Are you over 40?
Are you overweight?
Do you have any close relatives
with diabetes?

If you answered "yes" to any of these questions, you are at risk for diabetes. Close to 11 million Americans have diabetes. This number, growing by 8 percent each year, is expected to rise dramatically as the baby boomers (those born between 1946 and 1964) reach their forties. This group of 76 million is *one third of the entire U.S. population.* That means at least one out of three Americans is at risk for diabetes.

THE DIABETES CARBOHYDRATE AND CALORIE COUNTER

ANNETTE B. NATOW, Ph.D., R.D., and JO-ANN HESLIN, M.A., R.D., are the authors of ten books on nutrition, including *The Cholesterol Counter, The Fat Counter,* and *The Fat Attack Plan* (all available from Pocket Books). Both are former faculty members of Adelphi University and State University of New York, Downstate Medical Center. They are editors of the *Journal of Nutrition for the Elderly,* serve as editorial board members for the *Environmental Nutrition Newsletter,* and are frequent contributors to magazines and journals.

Books by Annette B. Natow and Jo-Ann Heslin

The Antioxidant Vitamin Counter
The Cholesterol Counter
The Diabetes Carbohydrate and Calorie Counter
The Fast-Food Nutrition Counter
The Fat Attack Plan
The Fat Counter
The Iron Counter
Megadoses
No-Nonsense Nutrition for Kids
The Pocket Encyclopedia of Nutrition
The Pregnancy Nutrition Counter
The Sodium Counter
The Supermarket Nutrition Counter

Published by POCKET BOOKS

The
DIABETES
CARBOHYDRATE
& CALORIE
COUNTER

Annette B. Natow, Ph.D., R.D.,
and Jo-Ann Heslin, M.A., R.D.

POCKET BOOKS

New York   London   Toronto   Sydney   Singapore

An *Original* Publication of POCKET BOOKS

POCKET BOOKS, a division of Simon & Schuster Inc.
1230 Avenue of the Americas, New York, NY 10020

ISBN: 0-671-69565-7

First Pocket Books printing November 1991

10

POCKET and colophon are registered trademarks of Simon & Schuster Inc.

Front cover design by Raquel Jamarillo

Printed in the U.S.A.

To our families who support us through every project:
Harry, Allen, Irene, Sarah, Meryl, Laura,
Marty, George, Emily,
Steven, Joseph, Kristen and Karen

ACKNOWLEDGMENTS

Without the tireless cooperation of Steven, *The Diabetes Carbohydrate and Calorie Counter* would never have been completed. Our thanks to Dr. Martin Lefkowitz, Dr. Irene Rosenberg, Alma Flaumenhaft, and David H. Raab, Ph.D., for reviewing the material. We appreciate the generosity of the American Diabetes Association and the pharmacy department of Mercy Hospital, Rockville Centre, in sharing resources. A special thanks to our agent, Nancy Trichter, and Sally Peters, our editor.

"The regulation of the diet is the most important consideration in the treatment of diabetes mellitus."

"While certain general principles in regard to diet for diabetes can be laid down, each patient presents an individual problem. . . ."

Mary Swartz Rose, Ph.D.
Feeding the Family
The Macmillan Company, 1919

CONTENTS

3

SUGAR BASICS
35

4

INDIVIDUALIZING YOUR EATING PLAN
41

5

USING THE DIABETES COUNTER
84

THE DIABETES CARBOHYDRATE
AND CALORIE COUNTER
87

PREFACE

Diabetes is a condition that requires many lifestyle changes in order for medical treatment to be successful. People with diabetes, therefore, must become personally involved in their treatment. It is not enough just to take medicine; proper diabetes management requires careful attention to the meal plan, exercise, and diabetes monitoring, in addition to merely "taking the medicine."

Due to this unique condition, the person with diabetes is not just a recipient of medical care. He or she is an active participant in it.

In order for someone to effectively participate in his or her own health care, education about how to treat diabetes is essential. Still, making some of the required adjustments may not be easy. It helps for the person with diabetes to understand why such changes are needed, rather than mechanically following a doctor's instructions.

In *The Diabetes Carbohydrate and Calorie Counter*, Annette B. Natow and Jo-Ann Heslin provide explanations for these necessary changes in dietary habits. The authors have combined two aspects that are essential to treatment success: *what* you need to do, and *why* you need to do it.

In an accessible style, even to those without a medical background, Natow and Heslin provide the rationale for the diabetic meal plan grounded in an understanding of the mechanisms that cause diabetes. They then give logical recommendations for an eating program based on this foundation.

Finally, Natow and Heslin provide the tools for daily adherence to a medical program. Although willpower can be difficult to control, the authors' suggestions will assist those who wish to make an effort to change their lives and follow the guidelines of a health-care team.

As a supplement to an overall diabetes treatment program instituted by a health-care team (which should include a dietitian), *The Diabetes Carbohydrate and Calorie Counter* is a useful tool for anyone who wishes to treat his or her diabetes with precision and understanding.

Richard S. Beaser, M.D.,
Chief, Patient Education
Joslin Diabetes Center

The
DIABETES
CARBOHYDRATE
& CALORIE
COUNTER

1

UNDERSTANDING DIABETES

STAYING HEALTHY

Are you over forty?
Are you overweight?
Do you have any close relatives with diabetes?

If you answered "yes" to any of these questions, you are at risk for diabetes. Diabetes or, more accurately, diabetes mellitus is a common, chronic problem found throughout the world. Close to 11 million Americans have it, but many don't even know they do.

Anne R., a 47-year-old salesclerk who weighed more than she should, went to the doctor for an examination for a vaginal infection. The doctor treated her problem and found a second one. Anne was diabetic.

Tom O. visited his eye doctor for a checkup after failing the routine eye examination for renewal of his driver's license. While examining his eyes, the doctor suggested that Tom see his family doctor who, in turn, diagnosed diabetes.

Anne and Tom, like many other healthy people, were unaware of the early warning symptoms for diabetes. Recurrent vaginal infections and vision changes are two early signs. (See the highlight box "Warning Signs for Diabetes," page 2.)

WARNING SIGNS FOR DIABETES

Increased thirst
Frequent urination
Unintended weight loss
Blurred vision
Numbness or tingling in arms or legs
Frequent infections
Slow-healing cuts and bruises
Drowsiness
Fatigue
Diarrhea

Most people have one or more of these symptoms at some time or other. They are often ignored or simply considered part of getting older. Some people with diabetes have no symptoms at all and the condition may be discovered during a routine checkup.

The number of people with diabetes is growing by 8 percent each year. This is expected to rise dramatically as the baby boomers, those born between 1946 and 1964, reach their forties. This group numbers 76 million or *one third of the entire U.S. population*. That means at least one out of three Americans is at risk for diabetes.

After age forty, the incidence of diabetes increases. By age sixty-five, there is a 50 percent chance of developing it. That's why it's important that everyone have an understanding of this all-too-common problem.

Diabetes seems to run in families. If you have a close relative—a parent, grandparent, uncle, aunt—who has diabetes, you may be in danger of getting it too. But just because you carry the genetic trait for diabetes doesn't mean you will become diabetic. Many people who are potential diabetics never get it. Many things can be done to protect yourself. The best defense against the most common form of diabetes is to stay slim.

Being overweight increases your risk. How much you eat and what you eat are both important in preventing health problems. A healthy preventive diet is one that:

- has enough calories to maintain your best weight
- is low in total fat
- is low in saturated fat
- is low in sweets
- is moderate in protein
- is high in starch
- is high in fiber

APPLE OR PEAR?

To find out which shape you are:

1. Using a tape measure, measure around your waist where it's smallest. Measure while you are relaxed; don't pull in your stomach.
2. Measure around your hips at the widest part.
3. Divide the waist measurement by the hip measurement to get your result.

Women with figures below 0.75 are pears; above 0.85 are apples. Apples are at greater risk.

Men with figures below 0.80 are pears; above 0.95 are apples. Apples are more common in men and indicate greater risk.

You can lower your hip to waist ratio when you lose weight.

HOW DIABETES GOT ITS NAME

Diabetes has been around for a long time. Writings in ancient civilizations in Egypt, Greece, Rome and India described its symptoms. It was noted that people with the disorder passed large amounts of honey-sweet urine, which attracted ants and flies. Indian writings blamed overeating, and the Egyptians recommended a diet of beer, fruits, grains and honey.

A Roman named the condition *diabetes*, meaning "to flow through," because of the frequent thirst and urination often associated with it. In 1675, a London physician added the term *mellitus*, which is Latin for "honeylike," describing the sweet taste of the urine. *Diabetes mellitus* is the accurate name for the condition simply called diabetes.

Your body shape is as important as how much you weigh. Look at yourself in the mirror. Do you look like an apple or a pear? If you have excess fat around your middle, you are apple-shaped and at greater risk for diabetes and other serious health problems. Do you carry your fat around your hips and on your thighs? If so, you are considered to be pear-shaped and at less risk of developing diabetes and other serious problems.

UNDERSTANDING DIABETES

Most people think that a person with diabetes can't eat sugar, but the problem is much more complex than that. The diabetic person cannot efficiently use the energy (calories) found in foods. The foods we eat contain energy in the form of protein, fat and carbohydrate. After being eaten, foods are broken down in the digestive tract and are then absorbed by the body's cells. Energy is finally released in the cell, so the breakdown products of food eaten must get inside the cell. That's the problem in diabetes. Digested food cannot be moved into the cell.

A hormone, *insulin,* is the carrier that helps potential energy enter the cell. Insulin is produced by specialized cells in the pancreas, a gland just below and behind the stomach. Some people do not make enough insulin while others make enough or even too much.

When a person's pancreas produces too little insulin, the result is obvious: Needed fuel cannot enter the cell. Others, who make the right amount of insulin or too much insulin, have another problem: Something prevents the body from using this insulin.

The result of either too little insulin or ineffective insulin is the same. Fuel does not get into the cell.

What Really Happens

The body uses glucose (sugar) and fat as fuel. The process involved in converting glucose and fat into energy is very complicated. Carbohydrates—starches and sugars found in milk, fruit, potatoes, breads and other foods—are easily broken down to glucose. The glucose can be used immediately for fuel or it can be changed into glycogen (storage fuel) and stored in the liver and muscles for future use. Any glucose not needed for fuel or for glycogen is changed into fat and stored in the body. This fat can, at some future time, be changed back into glucose.

Fat—found in foods like butter, margarine, oils, nuts, meat and other foods—is another form of fuel. When fat is digested, fatty acids are formed. Insulin helps the fatty acids enter fat cells, where they are stored for future use as fuel.

Protein—found in meat, fish, poultry, cheese, milk, beans and other foods—is made up of amino acids, the building blocks of protein. When protein is digested, the result is amino acids. Some of these amino acids may be changed into glucose in the liver. This happens when there is not enough carbohydrate to use for fuel.

Now you can see why insulin is so important. Insulin helps the body use all types of food energy—carbohydrate, fat and protein. It helps in the storage of carbohydrate, fat and protein by increasing the movement of glucose, fatty acids and amino acids into the cells. It also stimulates the building of protein, glycogen and fat in the body. The net effect of all this is reduced blood sugar (glucose) levels.

Normally, when food is eaten, enough insulin is produced to take care of all these functions. In diabetes, when there is either too little insulin or the insulin does not work well, sugar (glucose) accumulates in the blood. It can be as high as 300 to 1200 mg/dl (milligrams of sugar per deciliter of blood). The normal fasting level is 80 to 120 mg/dl. "Fasting" refers to abstaining from eating for 8 to 12 hours. Before a routine blood test a person is usually required to abstain from eating overnight. (See the highlight box "Terms Used to Measure Blood Sugar," page 7.) A higher than normal blood sugar level is called *hyperglycemia* (*hyper*=high, *glyc*= glucose, *emia*=in the blood).

In hyperglycemia, sugar builds up in the blood and circulates through the kidneys. Usually, when the blood sugar level rises over 180 mg/dl, the kidneys cannot handle that much sugar. The extra sugar is passed out of the body in the urine. Sugar found in the urine is a sign that something is wrong.

Sometimes, in older people, there may be no sugar in the urine even though the blood sugar level is higher than 180 mg/dl. This is because, in some people, the kidneys may work less efficiently as they age. In these cases, diabetes is confirmed through a blood test. That is one reason why your doctor orders a blood test during your annual physical.

TERMS USED TO MEASURE BLOOD SUGAR

mg = milligram
dl = deciliter

Blood sugar is measured in milligrams (mg). A milligram is one thousandth of a gram. To put that in perspective, there are approximately four grams of sugar in a teaspoon. A milligram equals 1/4000 of a teaspoon. A deciliter (dl) is one tenth of a liter, or a little less than one-half cup. The number of milligrams of sugar in a deciliter of blood is the ratio used to measure the sugar level of the blood.

For example, a blood sugar level of 120 mg/dl means that there are 120 milligrams of sugar in a deciliter of blood.

Another way to express the same measurement is 120 mg %. You may see this measurement on the results of your blood test.

TYPES OF DIABETES

There are two main types of diabetes. The most common and the one that this book focuses on is Type II. Ninety percent of all people with diabetes have this form of the disorder.

Type II (NIDDM)

Type II diabetes used to be called maturity-onset or adult-onset diabetes because most people developed it after age forty. Type II may also be called *non-insulin-dependent diabetes mellitus* or NIDDM. This is because most people with this type of diabetes do not need to take insulin, although about one third will need insulin at some point in their lives.

In Type II diabetes, the pancreas continues to function, but either too little insulin is produced or the insulin that is made is not used effectively. Body cells may resist the insulin.

Eighty percent of the people who have Type II diabetes are overweight when the condition is diagnosed. Fat cells are insulin resistant and may prevent the body from using insulin normally. That's why being overweight is an important factor for Type II diabetes. Even a person who is only moderately overweight increases his risk. Studies show that weighing only 20 percent more than desirable doubles the chance of developing diabetes.

It's surprising to learn that some people with Type II diabetes have normal or above normal amounts of insulin in their blood. It is believed that some of these people may have fewer receptor sites for insulin on their cells. These are the places where insulin can hook up and let glucose enter the cell. In other people, there are sufficient receptor sites, but the insulin does not stay hooked to the receptors. This is known as insulin resistance. In other words, these people are resistant to using their own insulin. In addition, a person who is overweight has increased insulin resistance.

For a newly diagnosed Type II diabetic, the most important goal is to lose weight. This is accomplished through diet and exercise. Developing healthy eating habits—less fat and sugar, more starch and fiber—and adopting an exercise program are the first steps in the treatment of diabetes. Together, diet and exercise achieve two things: weight is lost and blood sugar goes down.

Some people who are very resistant to their insulin may need to take insulin injections or diabetes pills (oral hypo-glycemic agents) until some weight is lost. (See the highlight box "Diabetes Pills and Insulin," page 9.) This may make it take longer to lose weight because both insulin and diabetes pills can increase the appetite. Persistence pays off, and even though weight comes off slowly, as fat is lost the body becomes more sensitive to its own insulin. At this point the insulin or diabetes pills are often no longer needed.

Losing weight doesn't cure Type II diabetes, but it can help control it. A person with Type II diabetes who loses weight and keeps it off may live a life free of diabetes-related

DIABETES PILLS AND INSULIN

DIABETES PILLS

Diabetes pills or oral hypoglycemic agents (OHAs) are used in Type II diabetes when weight loss, diet and regular exercise are not enough to keep blood sugar within a desirable range. Oral agents stimulate the body to use its own insulin. They do not work if the pancreas is not producing any insulin. That is why these pills are not useful for people with Type I diabetes. Oral hypoglycemic agents are not recommended for use during pregnancy or breastfeeding or by someone who is allergic to sulfur drugs.

Each person needs to have his physician individualize his treatment with OHAs.

INSULIN

Insulin injections may be needed in Type II diabetes when weight loss, healthy eating, exercise and even oral hypoglycemic agents are not enough to keep blood sugar levels within a desirable range.

Insulin is a hormone made in the pancreas that helps glucose get into the cells. In the past, insulin from the pancreas of a cow or a pig was given to diabetics. Today, human-type insulin is produced in a laboratory.

Because insulin is a protein, it cannot be taken by mouth. If swallowed, it would be digested and broken down to its amino acids (building blocks) and no longer function as a hormone. That's the reason why insulin is given as an injection.

Each person needs to have his insulin dose individualized by his physician.

problems. At the same time, healthy eating, exercise and maintaining normal weight help protect against other health risks: heart disease, high blood cholesterol, high blood pressure, certain cancers, gall bladder disease, gout, respiratory problems, arthritis and digestive problems.

Type I (IDDM)

Type I diabetes is the less common form of diabetes, with only about 10 percent of all diabetics falling into this group. Type I diabetes used to be called juvenile-onset because most people developed it during childhood or as young adults. The average age of onset is twelve, but a very small percentage of those with Type I diabetes develop it when they are older. It is often referred to as *insulin-dependent diabetes mellitus* or IDDM. This is because people with Type I diabetes do not produce any insulin at all. No one knows exactly why this happens, but some researchers believe that it may be because the body mistakenly attacks the insulin-producing cells of the pancreas and destroys them. (See the highlight box "What the Researchers Are Saying," page 11.) Other causes of Type I diabetes may be severe malnutrition, starvation or a serious disease that damages the pancreas. Those with Type I diabetes must have insulin injections every day.

Weight loss is a common early symptom of this form of diabetes because the body cannot use food normally without insulin. The result is the same as starvation. When there is no insulin, the body starts to burn its own body fat for the energy it needs. Whenever fat is burned for energy, *ketones* are formed as by-products. Without insulin, these ketones build up in the blood. This results in a serious condition called *ketoacidosis.* People with Type I diabetes must take insulin to avoid this life-threatening condition. This problem rarely occurs in people with Type II diabetes.

WHAT THE RESEARCHERS ARE SAYING

Researchers are on the way to discovering how to prevent one form of diabetes, Type I or *insulin-dependent diabetes mellitus* (IDDM). Type I diabetes is an autoimmune disorder. Only about 10 percent of all diabetics are Type I. Normally the body produces antibodies to fight foreign invaders like the bacteria that cause infections, but in the case of Type I diabetes the body makes antibodies that destroy its own tissue. An enzyme in the pancreas that seems to be the target of this misguided attack has been identified. Researchers have been able to use a blood test based on this enzyme to identify people who are on their way to developing Type I diabetes. In susceptible people, drugs that suppress immune function are being tried to see if they can stop the damage to the pancreas that sets the stage for Type I diabetes.

GESTATIONAL DIABETES (PREGNANCY-INDUCED DIABETES)

There is a special type of diabetes that occurs during pregnancy. Most women are able to produce enough insulin and use it normally until they are stressed by a pregnancy. During pregnancy, many women become temporarily insulin-resistant, but the problem disappears after the baby is born. Today, pregnant women are routinely tested for gestational diabetes. Early diagnosis and proper care can prevent medical problems for mother and baby.

Most women with gestational diabetes can control it by modifying their diet. Weight loss is *not* recommended during pregnancy, but for overweight women, losing weight after delivery may prevent a recurrence of gestational diabetes during their next pregnancy. Having gestational diabetes is a warning signal that a woman may be at greater risk of developing Type II diabetes later in life.

2

NUTRITION BASICS

UNDERSTANDING NUTRIENTS

At the end of 1990, after studying the relationship between diet and health, the U.S. Department of Agriculture and the Department of Health and Human Services released an update of the Dietary Guidelines for Americans. These guidelines are an answer to the question "What should Americans eat to stay healthy?" They are recommended for healthy Americans ages two and over. The advice is good for people with diabetes as well. In fact, you'll see that a few of the guidelines are the same as the ones recommended by the American Diabetes and Dietetic Associations. (See "Getting Started" in chapter 4, page 43.)

- Eat a variety of foods
- Maintain healthy weight
- Choose a diet low in fat, saturated fat and cholesterol
- Choose a diet with plenty of vegetables, fruits and grain products
- Use sugars only in moderation
- Use salt and sodium only in moderation
- If you drink alcoholic beverages, do so in moderation

These guidelines stress moderation in the use of sugar, salt, alcohol, fat, saturated fat and cholesterol. A healthy diet emphasizes vegetables, fruits and grains. What you eat is one of the most important factors both in good health and, most important, in diabetes care. The following sections will tell you all you should know about the different nutrients you need. This information will be valuable for planning your lifelong eating plan.

CALORIES AND WEIGHT

Calories are a measure of the energy or heat in food. The amount of energy that is needed to do the body's work is measured as the amount of heat produced by normal body activity—breathing, blood circulation, digesting food, growing, repairing damaged tissues (cuts, broken legs) and walking.

The energy value of food is measured in the calories that the food will produce when burned. We get calories when we eat carbohydrate, fat and protein in foods. One gram (about one-quarter teaspoon) of carbohydrate or protein has four calories. One gram of fat has nine calories. Alcohol contains calories too, seven in a gram.

When we eat more calories than are needed to supply the body with energy, the excess calories are converted to fat and stored for future use. This results in weight gain. When too few calories are eaten, stored fat is used for energy and weight is lost.

You may wonder how many calories you need each day. It's easy to figure this out.

How many calories do you need each day?

To answer this question, first you need to determine your desirable weight.

Suggested Weight for Adults

Height[1]	Weight In Pounds[2,3]	
	19 to 34 years	35 years and over
5'0"	97–128	108–138
5'1"	101–132	111–143
5'2"	104–137	115–148
5'3"	107–141	119–152
5'4"	111–146	122–157
5'5"	114–150	126–162
5'6"	118–155	130–167
5'7"	121–160	134–172
5'8"	125–164	138–178
5'9"	129–169	142–183
5'10"	132–174	146–188
5'11"	136–179	151–194
6'0"	140–184	155–199
6'1"	144–189	159–205
6'2"	148–195	164–210
6'3"	152–200	168–216
6'4"	156–205	173–222
6'5"	160–211	177–228
6'6"	164–216	182–234

[1] Without shoes.
[2] Without clothes.
[3] The higher weights in the ranges generally apply to men, who tend to have more muscle and bone; the lower weights more often apply to women, who have less muscle and bone.

Source: *Dietary Guidelines for Americans,* 3rd edition, 1990, USDA, USDHHS.

ESTIMATED DESIRABLE WEIGHT

Women: 100 pounds for first 5 feet of height. Add 5 pounds for each additional inch or subtract 5 pounds for each inch less than 5 feet.

Men: 106 pounds for first 5 feet of height. Add 6 pounds for each additional inch.

For both women and men, add 10 percent for a large body frame; subtract 10 percent for small body frame.

Example: Stephanie is 5 feet, 6 inches tall with an average frame.

```
   5 feet = 100 pounds
 6 inches =  30 pounds
            130 pounds
```

Example: Henry is 6 feet with a large body frame.

```
    5 feet = 106 pounds
 12 inches =  72 pounds
             178 pounds
           +  18 pounds (10% of 178 pounds for large
                         body frame)
             195 pounds
```

Another way to determine your desirable weight is to refer to "Suggested Weights for Adults," page 14, from the third edition of Dietary Guidelines for Americans.

Once you know your desirable weight you can determine your daily calorie needs.

To estimate daily calorie requirement:

Very active men
20 calories × your desirable body weight

Moderately active men or very active women
15 calories × your desirable body weight

Inactive men and all people over age 55
13 calories × your desirable body weight

Inactive women, very overweight people and repeat
dieters
10 calories × your desirable body weight

In *The Diabetes Counter* we often refer to "reasonable weight." This is the weight that an overweight person with Type II diabetes can hope to achieve. It may be slightly more than a calculated "Desirable Weight" as computed above.

CARBOHYDRATE (CHO)

Carbohydrates include sugars, starch and fiber. The sugars and starches are digested and converted into energy for the body to use. Excess carbohydrate is stored as fat. A small amount is stored as glycogen in the liver and muscles. Fiber cannot be digested and is not used by the body for energy.

Food that contains carbohydrate can raise the level of blood sugar. Glucose is a simple sugar (monosaccharide) found in the blood. A higher than normal level of glucose in the blood is a sign of diabetes. Another simple sugar is fructose, found in fruit. Ordinary table sugar is a combination of glucose and fructose, making a double sugar (disaccharide). Most sweeteners that we use—corn syrup, honey, maple syrup—are combinations of monosaccharides and disaccharides.

Starch, the way energy is stored in plants, is a larger sugar complex made up of many monosaccharides. Wheat, corn, rice, potatoes and beans are good sources of starch. The starch in foods must be broken down by digestion into glucose before it is absorbed.

Americans get more than 50 percent of their calories as carbohydrate. Carbohydrate foods are an important part of a diabetic eating plan too. In fact, most of the calories in the diabetic diet come from carbohydrate. People with Type II diabetes benefit from diets high in carbohydrate. These foods help maintain normal blood sugar levels. Sugar needs to be limited and should be eaten only at mealtimes.

The use of sugar is controversial. Experts recommend that no more than 5 percent of the total carbohydrate calories each day come from plain sugar. This would be two teaspoons on a 1500-calorie diet. That means that when you eat foods like desserts or cookies that were made with sugar (not artificial sweetener), you should eat only the amount of that food that contains one teaspoon of sugar. For example, if you make applesauce containing two tablespoons of sugar, you can eat one sixth of the recipe, as that would be the equivalent of one teaspoon of sugar. The sugar is used as a replacement for other carbohydrates and not as additional carbohydrate.

Even though small amounts of sugar are permitted in diabetic diets, it is important to carefully limit the amount of all sweeteners used. Too much sugar can use up the body's supply of chromium. The mineral chromium is needed for insulin to work properly. When a lot of monosaccharides (glucose and fructose) are eaten, they cause the body to waste chromium. You can conserve chromium by avoiding simple sugars.

Blood Sugar Index (Glycemic Index)

The common belief that sugar causes an immediate and greater increase in blood glucose levels than starch is not always true. All sugars do not have the same effect on blood sugar. Different kinds of carbohydrates, because of their varying structure, are absorbed by the body in different ways. Research in the last decade has shown that the effect of different foods on blood sugar depends on many things:

Is the food liquid or dry?
Is it finely ground or coarse?
How much fat, fiber and protein are in the food?
How digestible is the food?
Is the food completely cooked?

All of these factors working together produce a food's *glycemic index,* a relative measure of how quickly a carbohydrate food causes blood sugar to increase. Of all foods studied, legumes (peas, beans and especially lentils) have the least effect on blood glucose. Yogurt and milk come next, then fruits. Vegetables vary in their effect on blood sugar with parsnips, carrots and instant mashed potatoes raising blood sugar more than sweet potatoes and potato chips.

FOODS LEAST LIKELY TO RAISE BLOOD SUGAR LEVELS*

Apples	Oranges
Black-eyed peas	Pasta (white & whole wheat)
Cherries	Peanuts
Chickpeas	Pears
Dried green peas	Plums
Grapefruit	Skim milk
Ice cream	Soybeans
Kidney beans	Sweet potatoes
Lentils	Whole milk
Lima beans	Yogurt

*Foods are listed in alphabetical order, not according to their ability to raise blood sugar.

Pastas have less effect than either white or whole wheat bread.

The value of using the glycemic index in planning diabetic diets is controversial. However, the position of the American Diabetes Association is that diabetics should choose most frequently those carbohydrate-containing foods that are least likely to raise blood sugar levels.

Fiber

Fiber is the type of carbohydrate that cannot be digested. It's found in food from plants like whole grains, beans, fruits and vegetables. Fiber comes from different parts of plants:

leaves like spinach
stems like celery
flowers like broccoli
tubers like potatoes
roots like carrots
seeds like sunflower
grains like whole wheat

Americans are being urged to double the amount of fiber they eat. Some of the health benefits of fiber have been known for a long time. Roughage, another name for fiber, is an old remedy for constipation. More recently, it has been discovered that in areas of the world where people eat more fiber, diabetes, heart disease and certain types of cancer are less common.

Fiber may be of special importance in the diabetic diet. Research shows that eating fiber can help in three ways:

1. It keeps blood sugar levels from rising quickly after eating.

2. It helps decrease triglycerides and cholesterol levels in the blood.
3. It is bulky and so increases satiety (fullness); this helps weight loss.

There are actually two types of fiber: *soluble* and *insoluble*. Soluble fiber dissolves in water, while insoluble does not. Most foods from plants contain both kinds of fiber, but they usually have more of one type than the other. Both soluble and insoluble fiber fill you up and help weight loss but, aside from that, each one has specific health benefits.

Insoluble fiber helps relieve constipation by bulking up the stools. It acts like a sponge, absorbing water so stools get softer and move along the intestines more quickly. Vegetables, whole wheat and other whole grains like corn and rye are rich in insoluble fiber.

Soluble fiber helps keep blood sugar levels low and also reduces the amount of triglycerides and cholesterol in the blood. Citrus fruits, oats, barley, dried peas and beans are rich in soluble fiber.

It is recommended that people with diabetes eat more fiber. If diabetes pills or insulin are used, discuss adding fiber with your doctor. When you are eating more fiber, it is necessary to monitor blood sugar levels carefully. Increasing your fiber intake may require an adjustment in the amount of medication you take. When necessary, your doctor will help you with this.

When you begin to add high-fiber foods to your diet, be sure to drink plenty of liquids. Constipation can result when fiber is increased and fluids are not increased at the same time. Often, people experience bloating, diarrhea and gas when fiber intake is increased too quickly. Gradually increasing the amount of high-fiber foods eaten gives your body time to adjust and may prevent these discomforts.

HOW TO ADD FIBER

Choose a variety of:
  Whole-grain breads and cereals
  Unpeeled fruits and vegetables—raw whenever possible
  Dried peas and beans, lentils and barley

Start with one or two servings a day and increase gradually.
Drink six to eight glasses of liquids each day. Bran or fiber pills
are not necessary. It's healthier to get your fiber in food.

PROTEIN

Protein is part of every cell and substance in the body.
Protein in the food we eat provides the raw material to build
the body's tissues. Besides building and repairing the body,
protein can be used to make sugar (glucose) and provide
energy if there is not enough energy available from carbohydrate and fat.

Amino acids are the building blocks of protein. There are
over twenty different amino acids. Some of these amino
acids must be obtained directly from food, while others can
be made in the body. The assortment of amino acids that is
found in a particular protein determines its structure and
function. For example, hair is made of amino acids and so
are skin and blood, but the assortment of amino acids in
each is different.

Protein foods that come from animals—milk, cheese,
meat and eggs—are called high-quality proteins because
they contain the amino acids that cannot be made in the
body. Plant proteins—grains, beans, nuts—do not each con-

tain all the needed amino acids. When they are eaten together, as in a dish of rice and beans, the mixture of amino acids provided from the rice and beans supplies all that are needed.

Americans eat a lot of protein. Most of us get twice as much as we need. One problem with this excess is that animal proteins often come packaged with fat. Another possible problem, and this is controversial, is that too much protein could put a strain on the kidneys. This is because the kidneys must excrete the breakdown products of excess protein. In fact, some researchers believe that high-protein diets are responsible for reduced kidney function as people age. Kidney problems are more commonly found in people with diabetes. Diets for people with diabetes are usually planned to provide 15 to 20 percent of total calories in the form of protein.

FOODS HIGH IN PROTEIN

Cheese	Nuts
Dried peas and beans	Poultry
Eggs	Seeds
Fish	Tofu
Lentils	Whole-grain breads
Meat	and cereals
Milk	

FAT

Americans eat too much fat. It supplies about 37 percent of all the calories eaten each day. It would be healthier if fat provided no more than 30 percent of the calories. Fat is a concentrated source of calories; it contains, weight for weight, more than twice as many calories as carbohydrate or protein. That is why eating a lot of fat can make you fat.

But a small amount of fat is needed for good health. Besides calories, fat also provides essential fatty acids, which the body cannot make; it insulates the body, helping it to stay at a constant temperature; it protects vital organs like the kidneys, which are covered with fat; it carries fat-soluble vitamins (A, D, E, K) into the body; it's part of the membranes around cells; and just as important, fat makes foods taste good.

While it is true that a small amount of fat is necessary, too much is definitely unhealthy. High-fat diets raise the levels of triglycerides and fat in the blood, increasing the risk for heart attack and stroke. People with diabetes are at greater risk for heart disease, so lowfat diets should be a priority. Eating too much fat also increases the risk for breast, prostate and colon cancers, gallstones, gout and indigestion.

Fat Facts

Most of the fats in foods and in the body, too, are triglycerides. These triglycerides are made up of fatty acids plus glycerol. Depending on their chemical structure, the fatty acids are either saturated, polyunsaturated or monounsaturated.

All triglycerides contain a mixture of fatty acids. Fats are grouped according to the kinds of fatty acids they contain. When *most* of the fatty acids in a fat are:

saturated—the fat is "saturated"
polyunsaturated—the fat is "polyunsaturated"
monounsaturated—the fat is "monounsaturated"

For example, olive oil is called a monounsaturated fat because it contains *mainly* monounsaturated fatty acids. It also contains small amounts of polyunsaturated and saturated fatty acids. Safflower oil, on the other hand, is called a polyunsaturated fat because it contains more "polys" than other kinds of fatty acids.

Saturated Fats

Saturated fats stay solid at room temperature. Fat around a chop or steak is an example of saturated fat. Even if you left the meat on the kitchen counter for a few hours, the fat would still be solid.

Saturated fat usually comes from animal foods—meat, milk, cheese and butter. But some vegetable foods, mainly the tropical oils—coconut, palm, palm kernel—and cocoa butter are highly saturated too. When vegetable oils like corn oil are hardened (hydrogenated) to make margarine, they become more saturated.

As you probably know, saturated fats raise cholesterol levels in the blood. But recent studies show that not every saturated fat raises cholesterol. Beef, for example, contains several different saturated fats, among them palmitic fatty acid, which raises cholesterol, and stearic fatty acid, which lowers it. Foods have more than one type of saturated fatty acid. It's impossible to eat natural foods that contain only those saturated fatty acids that do not raise cholesterol.

Today, experts advise that your intake of saturated fats be limited to no more than one third (preferably 7 or 8 percent) of the 30 percent of calories allotted to fat. You can do this by eating less of the foods that are high in saturated fats. As these foods are often high in total fat as well, you will benefit twice—by reducing the intake of both saturated fat and total fat.

Later on in the book is a section that helps you plan your diet. You will select a calorie level to help you achieve your reasonable weight and you will keep track of calories and carbohydrates each day. Although you won't be keeping track of fat daily, it's wise to check the amount of fat you are eating. Once in a while, at least once a week, total the amount of fat in the foods you've selected for your daily meal plan. The fat figures provided in the counter will help make this an easy job. The following chart will give you the amount of fat, in grams, that will equal 30 percent of the calories as

THIRTY PERCENT FAT CALORIES

CALORIES	GRAMS OF FAT
1200	40
1500	50
1800	60
2100	70
2400	80
2700	90

FOODS HIGH IN SATURATED FATS

Beef	Hot dogs
Butter	Ice cream
Cheese	Lamb
Chicken	Lunch meats
Chocolate	Palm kernel oil
Coconut	Palm oil
Coconut oil	Pork
Cream	Sausage
Cream cheese	Sour cream
Duck	Veal
Fish	Whipped cream
Half & half	Whole milk

fat. For example, if you are on an 1800-calorie diet, you should eat approximately 60 grams of fat each day. This equals 30 percent of your day's total calories or a 30 percent fat diet.

Polyunsaturated Fats

Polyunsaturated fats are liquid at room temperature and remain liquid even when cold. Corn oil, for example, does not get solid even when refrigerated. Polyunsaturated fats may help lower cholesterol levels in the blood, but recent research suggests that too much polyunsaturated fat may not be good for your health. A diet high in polyunsaturated fats may cause gallbladder disease, depress the immune system and put you at greater risk for some cancers.

Fish contains unique polyunsaturated fats called EPA (eicosapentanoic acid) and DHA (docosahexanoic acid). They are often called omega-3 fatty acids or simply fish oils. These oils are found in larger amounts in fatty cold-water fish like salmon, mackerel, bluefish, herring, squid, rainbow trout and whitefish.

Studies have shown that fish-oil supplements may reduce the risk of heart disease, and are helpful in treating rheumatoid arthritis, high blood pressure, psoriasis, migraine headaches and in boosting immune function. Fish oils can also reduce triglyceride levels in people with elevated triglyceride levels in the blood.

Fish-oil supplements in capsule form were, until recently, available to consumers. Their use is controversial. In 1990, the Food and Drug Administration decided to stop the sale of fish-oil pills after concluding that they offer no known medical benefits.

Fish-oil supplements do not seem to help diabetes control in people with Type II diabetes. In two recent studies, fish-oil supplements reduced blood triglyceride levels, but worsened blood sugar control in poorly controlled Type II diabetics. Until more research is done to find out if fish-oil supplements are useful in diabetes, getting fish oils by eating more fish is a much better idea.

FOODS HIGH IN POLYUNSATURATED FATS

Bluefish	Sesame oil
Corn oil	Soft margarine
Cottonseed oil	Soybean oil
Herring	Sunflower oil
Mackerel	Tuna
Mayonnaise	Vegetable oil
Rainbow trout	Walnut oil
Sablefish	Walnuts
Safflower oil	Wheat germ
Salad dressing	Whitefish
Salmon	

Monounsaturated Fats

Monounsaturated fats are liquid at room temperature but become partly solid when chilled. Olive oil left out on the kitchen counter stays liquid, but it becomes cloudy (partly solid) when it is in the refrigerator. Monounsaturated fats can lower blood cholesterol when they are used in place of saturated fats. As a bonus, "mono's" are selective and lower the "bad" form of cholesterol (LDLs) and do not reduce the "good" form of cholesterol (HDLs). (See Cholesterol, page 28.) This is why it is recommended that more than one third of your daily fat intake come from monounsaturated fats. Some researchers are exploring the possible benefits of increasing monounsaturated fats in diabetic diets.

FOODS HIGH IN MONOUNSATURATED FATS

Almonds	Peanut oil
Canola oil	Peanuts
Cashews	Pine nuts (pignolia)
Chicken fat	Pistachio nuts
Filberts (hazelnuts)	Rice bran oil
Macadamia nuts	Sesame oil
Olive oil	Solid vegetable shortening
Olives	Soybean oil
Peanut butter	Soybean oil margarine

Cholesterol

Cholesterol is a white, waxy, fatlike substance that is part of every cell in your body. Cholesterol is necessary for body function. Hormones, nerve coverings, vitamin D, bile (used for digestion) and the fat that keeps your skin soft (sebum) are all made from cholesterol.

Although cholesterol is needed by the body, when the level of cholesterol in the blood gets too high, it increases your chances for heart disease. For adults, a level of more than 200 mg/dl is considered too high.

Because it is fatlike, cholesterol does not dissolve in the blood, which is mainly water. Instead it is transported by special lipoprotein carriers, which are little packages of fat wrapped in water-soluble protein. There are a few different carriers, but the two most important lipoproteins are listed here.

Low Density Lipoproteins (LDLs) are considered "bad" cholesterol because the cholesterol in LDLs can be deposited on your artery walls. High levels of LDLs (over 130 milligrams) are a risk factor for heart attacks and stroke.

High Density Lipoproteins (HDLs) are considered "good" cholesterol because they carry cholesterol back to the liver, where it is broken down and removed from the body. High levels of HDLs (over 45 milligrams for males, over 55 milligrams for females) are considered protective against heart attack and stroke.

All animal foods—meat, poultry, fish, eggs, milk, yogurt, cheese and butter—contain cholesterol. Egg yolks, caviar, liver and other organ meats like heart and brains are high in cholesterol. There is no cholesterol in food derived from plants, like fruits, vegetables, grains, beans, corn oil, peanut butter and nuts. Americans get about one third of their cholesterol from the foods they eat; the rest is made in the body.

Blood cholesterol levels are usually increased by the cholesterol, total fat and saturated fat that are consumed. High fiber intake may reduce cholesterol levels. Drinking more than three cups of coffee a day has been reported to increase cholesterol, while drinking tea, especially green tea (unfer-

---

FOODS HIGH IN CHOLESTEROL

American cheese	Ice Cream
Bacon	Kidney
Beef	Lamb
Brains	Liver
Butter	Pork
Caviar	Poultry
Cheddar cheese	Sardines
Cream	Sour cream
Cream cheese	Swiss cheese
Egg yolk	Veal
Fish	

---

mented), lowers it. Exercise and weight loss both lower cholesterol. High cholesterol also seems to run in families.

It is recommended that healthy adults eat no more than 300 milligrams of cholesterol a day. People with high blood cholesterol levels should have less—sometimes as little as 200 or 150 milligrams. Because people with diabetes are at greater risk for heart disease, they should keep the cholesterol in their diet low.

VITAMINS

Vitamins are chemicals that regulate the body's functions. They are vital to your life and health; you cannot live without them. Although vitamins do not give you calories (energy), they help turn the food eaten into useful energy. They also help the body grow and help nerves, muscles and organs work normally. You need only very small amounts of vitamins to do these jobs, sometimes as little as two micrograms. A microgram is one millionth of a gram. A teaspoon could hold four million micrograms!

Plants and animals make vitamins; we get most vitamins from foods from plants and foods from animals. We do, however, make very small amounts of some vitamins in our body: When skin is exposed to ultraviolet rays in sunlight, a fat in the skin is changed into vitamin D; bacteria that live in the intestines make vitamin K.

Vitamins are divided into two groups: *fat soluble,* those that dissolve in fat, and *water soluble,* those that dissolve in water. The fat soluble ones—A, D, E and K—are stored more easily in body fat. If an excess is taken as a supplement, these vitamins can accumulate over a period of time and become toxic to the body. Water soluble vitamins—C and the B vitamins—are more easily eliminated from the body, mainly in the urine.

Although vitamin C (ascorbic acid) is a water soluble vitamin and easily excreted from the body, taking large doses of the vitamin is not recommended for persons with diabetes. When a large amount of vitamin C is excreted in the urine, it can obscure the results of urine tests, giving false-positive results in some situations and false-negative results in others.

Large doses of one water soluble B vitamin, niacin, are used as a medication to help reduce blood cholesterol levels. Using three grams (3000 milligrams) daily has been shown to worsen diabetes. The RDA (Recommended Dietary Allowance) for niacin is 15 milligrams a day.

MINERALS

Minerals, like vitamins, act as regulators in the body. They are not a source of calories. They form part of body tissues, like the calcium found in bones and teeth. Or they may float in body fluids, like blood and tears, giving them their necessary characteristics. They are inorganic, smaller than vitamins and found in simple forms in foods.

Because the amounts of minerals found in and needed by the body vary, they are often subdivided into two categories: *major minerals* (macrominerals), which are needed in larger amounts, and *trace minerals* (microminerals), which are needed in smaller amounts.

Many minerals, such as iron, copper, magnesium, iodine and fluorine, are stored in the body and can be toxic when taken in excess. That is why it isn't a good idea to take supplements that provide more than RDA levels of minerals unless it has been suggested by your doctor.

Research suggests that adequate zinc intake may be helpful in preventing vision problems in people with diabetes. Getting zinc from foods rich in this mineral, like whole

CHROMIUM AND DIABETES

Chromium is a mineral needed by the body so that it handles carbohydrate and fat normally. It is part of the *glucose tolerance factor* (GTF) that helps insulin function. When there is a lack of chromium, the effectiveness of insulin is reduced. Some researchers believe that chromium deficiency may be a factor in Type II diabetes.

The intake of this mineral by most people is far less than the suggested safe and adequate range of 50 to 200 micrograms a day. In fact, the estimated intake is only one half of the 50 microgram minimum suggested.

Eating refined foods and those containing simple sugars aggravates the problem. These foods are low in chromium and deplete the body's supplies of the mineral when these foods are broken down and used. Besides high-sugar diets, strenuous exercise, physical trauma and infection also reduce the amount of chromium in the body.

As chromium is a nutrient and not a therapeutic agent, it will benefit only those people whose signs and symptoms of diabetes are due to marginal or more severe chromium deficiency. Chromium is found in all foods; meat, fish and fruit are the best sources. The amount of chromium in the soil determines the chromium level in foods grown in it and in animals that feed off the soil. Chromium in stainless-steel processing equipment and eating utensils and unlacquered, welded cans can leach out, increasing the level of chromium in the food with which they come in contact.

grains, meat and fish, is preferable to taking it in supplement form. Zinc supplements in amounts over the RDA may interfere with the body's use of the mineral copper.

Many studies point to the need for adequate chromium in people with diabetes. (See the highlight box "Chromium and Diabetes," above.)

Many experts feel that people on low-calorie diets may not be able to get all the needed vitamins and minerals from the small amount of food they eat. Taking a daily multi-vitamin/mineral supplement is wise. Select one with no more than 100 percent of the U.S. RDA.

FOODS HIGH IN CHROMIUM

The amount of chromium in the soil will determine the amount of the mineral in foods grown in it.

Egg yolks	Wheat germ
Fish	Whole grain cereals
Fruit	Whole grains
Meat	Yeast
Vegetable oils	

A WORD ABOUT ALCOHOL

Absolute abstinence is not necessary for most people with diabetes as long as the blood sugar level is controlled. Moderate amounts of alcohol taken before, during or immediately after eating will probably not affect blood sugar control.

Alcohol is a concentrated source of calories with no essential nutrients. One and a half ounces of 80 proof liquor contains about 100 calories as alcohol. Sweet wines, liqueurs and beer contain carbohydrates (and carbohydrate calories) in addition to alcohol. If you are overweight, these calories must be counted into your meal plan.

The American Diabetes Association recommends that alcohol be used only occasionally: one or two alcoholic drinks, once or twice a week. One alcoholic drink is equal to:

1½ ounces of whiskey, scotch, rye, vodka, gin, cognac, rum, dry brandy *or*
4 ounces of dry wine *or*
2 ounces of dry sherry *or*
12 ounces of light beer

Alcohol may cause problems with blood glucose control, increase triglycerides in the blood and interfere with the effectiveness of some drugs. This is why it is important that people with diabetes discuss using alcohol with their doctor.

3

SUGAR BASICS

SUGAR

Many people enjoy sweets. People with diabetes are better off indulging their "sweet tooth" with fruits—fresh, canned or dried. While it is best to avoid sugar, it may not always be possible. When you do eat a small amount of sugar, eat it at a meal to minimize its effect on blood sugar.

Sugar is a carbohydrate that provides four calories per gram, but it is not an essential food because it contributes few or no nutrients—vitamins, minerals or fiber. Its only contribution is calories. Most experts recommend that people with diabetes get no more than 5 percent of their calories from sugar.

To help you recognize less familiar sources of sugar in foods, see "Types of Sugars," below. To help you buy foods low in sugar see "Recognizing Sugar on Food Labels," page 37. See "Sugar-Free Over-the-Counter Medications," page 40, for a list of non-prescription drugs that do not have added sugar.

Types of Sugars

Brown Sugar A soft sugar in which the crystals are covered with a film of molasses syrup.

Corn sugar and syrup   A sugar made by the breakdown of cornstarch.

Dextrose   The commercial name for glucose.

Fructose   The simple sugar found in fruit, juices and honey.

Granulated sugar   The refined white sugar used as table sugar and in foods.

High-fructose corn syrup (HFCS)   The main sweetener used in processed foods and beverages—mostly fructose with some glucose.

Honey   Made by bees, this is an invert sugar with a little more fructose than glucose.

Invert sugar   Sugar broken down to glucose and fructose. It is sold as a liquid and used to keep baked goods and candies fresh.

Lactose   The sugar found in milk.

Maltose   A sugar formed by the breakdown of starch. Found in cereals and malted milk drinks.

Malto dextrins   Nonsweet sugars formed from the partial breakdown of starch. Used to improve texture and enhance flavor in candy, particularly chocolates.

Mannitol   Made from seaweed, it is used as a sweetner in foods, but it has calories and carbohydrates. Can cause digestive upset.

Maple sugar and syrup   Made by boiling down the sap of the sugar maple tree.

Molasses   The dark brown, thick syrup that is separated from raw sugar in the processing of white sugar.

Raw sugar   An unrefined sugar that may not be used in the U.S. until the impurities are removed.

Sorbitol   Used as a thickener in candy and as a sweetener in reduced-calorie foods. When eaten in excess it can cause diarrhea and gastrointestinal disturbance and can alter the absorption of drugs. Warning labels must appear on foods containing enough sorbitol that it is possible to eat more than 50 grams of sorbitol in one day.

Sorghum syrup   Mild, sweet syrup made from sorghum grain.

Sugar   See granulated sugar.

Turbinado sugar   Partially refined sugar with a tan to brown color.

Xylitol   A sugar that cannot be fermented by bacteria in the mouth, so it does not cause tooth decay. Used in chewing gum and mints. Large amounts can cause diarrhea.

RECOGNIZING SUGAR ON FOOD LABELS

WORDS ENDING IN -OSE	WORDS ENDING IN -OL
Dextrose	Mannitol
Fructose	Sorbitol
Glucose	Xylitol
Lactose	
Maltose	

OTHERS

Brown sugar	Malto dextrins
Corn sugar	Maple sugar
Corn sweetener	Maple syrup
Corn syrup	Molasses
High-fructose	Raw sugar
corn syrup	Sorghum
Honey	Turbinado sugar
Invert sugar	

SUGAR SUBSTITUTES

The American Diabetes Association has approved the use of low-calorie and calorie-free sugar substitutes for people with diabetes. These substitutes make it easier to stick to a healthy meal plan. Currently, there are three sugar substitutes approved for use: acesulfame-K (Sunette and Sweet One), aspartame (Nutrasweet or Equal) and saccharin. Sucralose, another sweetener, is close to being approved for use. The sweetener cyclamate was used in the 1960s until 1969, when it was taken off the market because it was believed to cause cancer. The FDA is considering a petition to reinstate approval of cyclamates.

Acesulfame-K

Two hundred times as sweet as sugar, acesulfame-K has been approved for use as a table sweetener and for powdered beverage mixes, gelatin puddings, chewing gum and non-dairy creamers. It contributes no calories because it is not broken down in the body. Acesulfame-K can also be used in baking.

Aspartame

Made up of two amino acids, aspartame is 180 times as sweet as sugar. There is only one calorie in the amount of aspartame equal in sweetness to one teaspoon of sugar. Aspartame cannot be used in cooking because its sweetness is lost when heated. This sweetener cannot be used by people with the inherited disorder PKU (phenylketonuria) and there is a warning about this on the labels of foods that contain aspartame.

Although there have been reports of dizziness and headaches from aspartame, repeated testing has shown the sweetener is safe when not used in excessive amounts. The FDA suggests that no more than 50 milligrams per kilogram (2.2 pounds) of body weight should be consumed daily. This is equal to about fourteen cans of diet soda a day for an adult.

Saccharin

Saccharin was the first man-made sugar substitute. It is 300 times as sweet as sugar. It provides no calories because it is not broken down in the body. It passes out of the body in urine unchanged. The government is currently reviewing the safety of saccharin. Results to date show the sweetener is safe to use. Until scientists complete their review of saccharin, all products that contain the sweetener must have a warning label.

Twenty milligrams of saccharin equal the sweetness of a teaspoon of sugar. An average diet soda sweetened with saccharin contains 150 milligrams of saccharin. It is often combined with other low-calorie sweeteners to mask its bitter aftertaste.

SUGAR IN MEDICATIONS

You may be surprised to learn that sugar is added to many common medications. This can create a problem in blood sugar control. There are many "sugar-free" over-the-counter medications. These "sugar-free" products may contain sorbitol, alcohol or other sources of carbohydrate even though they do not contain any sugar. Because manufacturers often change the formulas of their products, labels should be checked for the current listing of ingredients.

SUGAR-FREE OVER-THE-COUNTER MEDICATIONS

Centrafree Tablets
Chlor-Trimetron Tablets
Chloraseptic Mouthwash & Gargle
Chloraseptic Throat Spray
Chlorophyll Tablets
Cod Liver Oil (different brands)
Colace Liquid
Correctol Powder
Di-Gel Liquid
Dimetapp Elixir
Fiberall Natural Flavor Powder
Fiberall Orange Flavor Powder
Gaviscon Liquid
Gelucil-II Tablets
Gelucil-M Liquid
Gelucil-M Tablets
Gelucil Liquid
Gelucil Tablets
Geritol Complete Tablets
Haley's M-O
Maalox Plus Suspension
Maalox Plus Tablets
Maalox Suspension
Metamucil Sugar-Free Powder

Milk of Magnesia USP (different brands)
Mylanta II Liquid
Mylanta II Tablets
Mylanta Liquid
Mylanta Tablets
Mylicon Drops
One-A-Day Essential Tablets
Oyst-Cal 500 Tablets
Oystercal 500 Tablets
Pepto-Bismol Chewable Tablets
Pepto-Bismol Suspension
Riopan Plus Suspension
Riopan Suspension
St. Josephs Aspirin-Free Liquid
Sucrets Maximum Strength Mouthwash & Gargle
Tempra Tablets
Therevim Tablets
Tolu-Sed Cough Syrup
Tussex
Unicap Capsules or Tablets
Unicap-M

4

INDIVIDUALIZING YOUR
EATING PLAN

THE DIABETES DIET: PAST AND PRESENT

In 1550 B.C., an Egyptian remedy offered to "drive away the passing of too much urine" was a diet of beer, fruit, grains and honey. Indian writings from the same time stated that the disorder was due to overeating and excessive drinking. It is interesting to see that although diet treatments for diabetes have varied over the years—from high carbohydrate, to starvation, to low carbohydrate/high fat—we've come full circle to the very early Egyptian recommendation of high carbohydrate.

There is no single "diabetic diet." All are planned to help achieve reasonable weight, keep blood sugar and blood fat levels as close to the desirable range as possible, and provide all the nutrients needed to stay healthy. This is a good diet for everyone, diabetic or not.

A starting point for planning this healthy diabetic diet is the recommendations of The American Diabetes Association. They endorse a diet that provides about:

55% to 60% of calories as carbohydrates
12% to 20% of calories as protein
Less than 30% of calories as fat

Monounsaturated fats should make up the majority of fat in your diet. Cholesterol and salt should be limited while the amount of fiber should be increased.

The diet recommendations are straightforward and the benefits of following this healthy diet are proven. In spite of this, many people with Type II diabetes do not follow the dietary recommendations. In one survey, 80 percent of people with diabetes said they had received a written diet, but only 53 percent were using it. There are many reasons for this When faced with a lifetime of following a rigid diet "prescription," many people feel overwhelmed. It seems restrictive. While they are taught specifically what to eat—and what to avoid—they may not understand why.

Most people have some acquaintance with the nutrients—fat, carbohydrate, protein—found in foods. Food advertisements often emphasize these nutrients. Terms like "high protein," "lowfat," "high carbohydrate," "low cholesterol" are familiar. Some experts believe that the nutrient approach that is used to teach good nutrition may also be useful in helping people with diabetes follow healthy eating plans. A recent study that compared nutrient evaluation with traditional diet counseling in people with Type II diabetes found that a diet guide based on nutrients instead of foods was an effective way to help them follow a healthy diabetic eating plan.

The Diabetes Counter helps you do this. You have 3000 common foods, in usual portion sizes, along with the calories, carbohydrate and fat content. Foods high in sugar are noted with an asterisk. This is the information you need to plan a lifetime of healthy eating that will help control your diabetes. This diet plan can be tailored to meet special likes and dislikes. It is an individualized approach to healthy eating.

GETTING STARTED

The American Diabetes Association and the American Dietic Association agree on three nutritional goals for diabetes care. They recommend that people with diabetes achieve:

1. Appropriate blood glucose (sugar) and blood fat levels
2. Reasonable weight
3. Good nutrition

In simpler terms, these nutritional goals equal good, healthy eating for everyone. Only one goal—achieving appropriate blood glucose levels—is specific for people with diabetes. It is important to keep blood sugar levels as close to normal as possible. This helps prevent problems that can result when blood sugar gets too high. The less the blood sugar strays from the normal range, the more likely the body will stay healthy for many years.

Blood sugar levels in the body are controlled by a number of things, the three most important being *food eaten, activity* and *insulin*.

Eating and Activity

The amount of food eaten must be matched with the amount of insulin in the body. It doesn't matter if this insulin is produced in the body on its own, or if it is produced with the help of diabetes pills or if the insulin is injected. One way to make sure the food eaten matches the available insulin is to eat regular meals plus an optional snack near bedtime. Daily snacking is not necessary for most people with Type II diabetes. Weight control is the primary goal for those with Type II diabetes, and the calories eaten as a snack need to be counted toward their total calories for the day. In addition, it is important to go easy on sweets. These foods are often high in calories and fat as well. They are not good choices for people who need to lose weight, and they may outstrip the available insulin.

People with diabetes have a greater risk of developing heart disease. Heart attacks and strokes are major causes of death in the U.S. High levels of fats like cholesterol and triglycerides in the blood are risk factors for heart disease. That is why it is very important to eat a heart-healthy diet. This means eating foods that are low in total fat, saturated fat and cholesterol.

Weighing too much is not healthy for anyone, but it is especially bad for people with diabetes. As many as 40 percent of Americans weigh more than they should. Being overweight increases the risk for diabetes; it also worsens diabetes while at the same time increasing the risk for high blood pressure and heart disease.

Eating the right number of calories helps you reach and maintain a reasonable weight. The number of calories you need depends on your *age, size* and *activity.*

After age twenty-five, when you are fully grown, calorie needs go down gradually as you get older. This is due to changes in the body and the fact that people tend to be less active as they get older. People with a large body size need more calories than people with smaller frames. Simply moving a larger body around uses up more calories. The more active a person is, the more calories used. Walking uses more calories than sitting. And walking while carrying a heavy bag of groceries uses up even more calories.

Increased exercise is an important factor in good health and a way to reach and maintain a reasonable weight. Exercise has many other health benefits too: it helps lower blood sugar, triglycerides, and cholesterol; it reduces body fat; it strengthens the heart, muscles and bones; it even helps reduce stress.

Many people think that exercise must be vigorous and done for long periods of time to be beneficial. That is simply not true. Gradually increasing your activity at different times throughout the day is all you need to do. Even a few minutes of walking several times a day adds up. Walking is a wonderful exercise. Try climbing stairs instead of taking the elevator. Swimming, tennis and bicycling are all healthy and fun. If you do very little exercise, it's a good idea to check with your doctor before you begin any exercise program.

Individualized Care

Even though all people with Type II diabetes are often lumped together in one category, staying healthy is easier when care is individualized. To control blood sugar, an eating plan must be individually tailored to mesh with each person's lifestyle. Factors that affect eating—rest, exercise, relaxation, work schedule, smoking, support network—must all be considered. The last of these, the support network, should not be underestimated. Each person's habits and beliefs are shaped by family, friends and significant others. Eating is a social activity, often shared with others.

If weight loss is needed, this will be the primary focus. A person with newly diagnosed diabetes needs to relearn the art of eating: what to eat, when to eat and how to eat. For people with Type II diabetes, learning to eat the right amount of healthy foods may be all that is needed to control blood sugar levels.

This may sound easy but setting up your diabetic eating plan is a way of establishing good eating habits for the rest of your life. This is very different from a short-term diet designed to lose a few pounds. For the short term you are willing to accept a very limited diet. But when you are facing a lifelong "diet," you need an eating plan you can live with.

As you set up your diabetic eating plan, never forget that

eating is fun. Food is a source of comfort, enjoyment and pleasure as well as a vital source of calories and nutrients.

Your 55 Percent CHO (Carbohydrate) Eating Plan

To set up your 55 percent CHO eating plan you need to:

1. Determine your reasonable weight
2. Find out the number of calories you need each day to achieve or maintain your reasonable weight
3. Find out the daily amounts of carbohydrate on your 55 percent eating plan
4. Choose the foods you want to eat each day

Let's go through the process of setting up your eating plan one step at a time.

Reasonable Weight

Reasonable weight has no precise definition. It may be slightly more than desirable weight as calculated but falls within the range of suggested weights. It is the weight you can *reasonably* expect to reach and maintain comfortably. Most experts agree that weight loss, even a modest one, is helpful in controlling diabetes. Your overall goal is to lose weight even if it's only a small amount. For example, a 5'4" woman who weighed 160 pounds and reduced to 140 has achieved a reasonable weight. A 5'10" man who weighs 205 pounds weighs too much. See "Suggested Weight for Adults," page 14, and "Estimated Desirable Weight," page 14, to determine your reasonable weight goal.

Your Reasonable Weight is _____.

Number of Calories

When you have determined your reasonable weight, just multiply the weight as follows:

Very active man
   20 calores × reasonable body weight

Active men or very active women
   15 calories × reasonable body weight

Inactive men, moderately active women, all people over age 55
   13 calories × reasonable body weight

Inactive women, very overweight people, and repeat dieters
   10 calories × reasonable body weight

By using your reasonable body weight as the basis for figuring out the calories you need, you will automatically be choosing the right number of calories to help you reduce if you are overweight. A deficit of 500 calories a day will result in the loss of about one pound a week.

The 5'4", 140-pound woman who is moderately active will multiply 140 pounds by 13 calories to give her a daily calorie level of 1820 calories. This is enough to maintain her reasonable weight.

The 205-pound man who is overweight will find his reasonable weight by choosing a weight close to the upper limit of the range for his height, 5'10", from the chart "Suggested Weight for Adults," page 14. The suggested weight range is 146 to 188. Men fall in the upper limit of this range; 185 pounds would be considered reasonable for a 5'10" man. Being overweight, he multiplies this weight by 10 calories per pound, giving 1850 calories. At 205 pounds,

eating this calorie level daily will promote weight loss down
to approximately 180 pounds.

Now multiply your reasonable weight by the number of
calories per pound that you need for your activity level.

Reasonable weight × _____ calories.

Your daily calorie need is _____.

Carbohydrate Need

When you have determined your calorie needs, look in the
"55 Percent CHO (Carbohydrate) Eating Plan" chart to find
out how much carbohydrate you can have each day. If your
calorie level is not listed in the chart, choose the one that is
closest to yours. It's best to go down a few calories rather
than up.

---

55 PERCENT CHO (CARBOHYDRATE) EATING PLAN

CALORIES	CARBOHYDRATE (grams)
1200	165
1500	206
1800	248
2100	289
2400	330
2700	371

You can see that a person who needs 1800 calories a day
should have 248 grams of carbohydrate. For people who do
not take insulin or diabetes pills, the calories and carbohydrates will be divided into three meals a day plus one snack.
For example, breakfast can include about 20% of the calories, lunch 35%, dinner 35% and the snack 10%. For intakes

of 2400 calories or more, the calories and carbohydrates are distributed differently because additional snacks are included. See "Calorie and Carbohydrate Distribution for the Day," below.

The carbohydrate grams will be your guide to meal planning. It is best to have carbohydrate foods and calories distributed throughout the day.

CALORIE AND CARBOHYDRATE DISTRIBUTION FOR THE DAY

		B	L	D	S	S	S
1200	(C)	240	504	504	120	—	—
165	(CHO)	33	58	58	17	—	—
1500	(C)	300	525	525	150	—	—
206	(CHO)	41	72	72	21	—	—
1800	(C)	360	630	630	180	—	—
248	(CHO)	50	87	87	25	—	—
2100	(C)	420	735	735	210	—	—
289	(CHO)	58	101	101	29	—	—
2400*	(C)	480	720	720	240	240	—
330	(CHO)	66	99	99	33	33	—
2700*	(C)	540	675	675	270	270	270
371	(CHO)	74	93	93	37	37	37

C   = calories   B = Breakfast   D = Dinner
CHO = carbohydrates   L = Lunch   S = Snack

*Most people at these calorie levels find it more practical to divide their calories and carbohydrates into 3 meals and 2 or 3 snacks a day. The majority of people with Type II diabetes do not need this many calories a day unless they are very active.

People who take insulin injections may achieve better control with three meals plus three snacks a day—one at mid-morning and one at mid-afternoon in addition to one at bedtime. A similar food distribution is often recommended for people who take diabetes pills.

People who are taking insulin shots or diabetes pills should consult with their doctor, dietitian or diabetes educator to discuss how to divide the calories and carbohydrates into meals and snacks appropriate to their lifestyle and condition.

EATING WELL

How can you tell if you are meeting all your nutrient needs? One easy, effective way is to check your meal plans against the familiar Four Food Groups. When you eat the number of servings suggested for each of the four groups, you can be fairly certain that you are getting at least minimum amounts of all the nutrients you need.

Four Food Groups

Milk and Milk Products—2 servings a day. The major contribution of this group is the mineral calcium. This group includes milk, yogurt and cheese. Choose lowfat varieties whenever possible. A serving equals 1 cup of milk or yogurt or 1 ounce of cheese.

Breads and Cereals—4 or more servings a day. The major contributions of this group are energy, B vitamins and fiber. This group includes bread, rolls, bagels, cereals, pasta, rice, noodles, tortillas, pancakes. Choose whole grains whenever possible. A serving equals 1 slice of bread *or* 1 cup of cereal *or* ½ cup of pasta, noodles or rice.

Vegetables and Fruit—5 or more servings a day. The major contributions of this group are vitamins and minerals. This group includes all fruits and vegetables. A serving equals 1 cup raw *or* ½ cup cooked.

Meat and Meat Alternatives—6 to 8 ounces a day. The major contributions of this group are protein and the minerals iron and zinc. This group includes meat, poultry, fish, tofu, eggs, peas, beans, peanut butter. Choose lean foods whenever possible. A serving equals 3 to 4 ounces of meat *or* ½ cup of peas or beans *or* 2 tablespoons of peanut butter.

Three ounces of boneless meat, fish or poultry equal the size and thickness of a deck of cards.

These food groups are the foundation of your diet. Other foods like cream cheese, butter, desserts and alcohol can be used when calories permit.

SETTING UP YOUR EATING PLAN

Following are examples of a typical day's eating plan at the six different calorie levels. Keep track of the amount of calories and carbohydrate for each meal and snack. The six meal plans contain nutritious common foods that stay within the calorie and carbohydrate limits and meet all nutrient needs. Along with each eating plan is a blank worksheet. You can copy these worksheets to set up your individual eating plan.

As you fill in the worksheet, you'll see your calorie and carbohydrate targets for each meal on the left. When you have planned your meal and listed the food, portion, calories and carbohydrate, write the subtotals in the blanks at the right of the worksheet. Do this for each meal and snack throughout the day. Finally, total the entire day to see if it matches the targets for your eating plan.

It's not easy to plan a day's worth of meals that meet an exact number of calories and carbohydrates. Try to come as close as possible to the targets for each meal. You don't have to hit the target exactly.

At the bottom of the meal plan worksheets, you'll see the following footnotes: calories for a meal can be plus 25 or minus 25 calories; carbohydrate for a meal can be plus 5 or minus 5 carbohydrate grams.

The footnotes mean that you have a leeway of plus or minus 25 calories and plus or minus 5 carbohydrates at each meal or snack. By staying within these guidelines, you will be dividing your calories and carbohydrates throughout the day. By not eating too much at one time, you make it easier for your body to handle the food with the insulin available. This is the key to good control in a diabetic diet.

Meal Planning Hints

DO: Eat regular meals
       Choose suggested servings from the Four Food
          Groups
       Choose foods high in carbohydrate (starch) and fiber
       Choose foods low in fat
       Eat moderate amounts of all foods

Go Easy: On foods containing sugar
          On foods containing saturated fat
          Using alcohol

Don't: Skip meals
         Overeat

1200-Calorie Eating Plan

A 1200-calorie eating plan is very restrictive. It's best to stay at this calorie level for one month to achieve quick weight loss. Then move up to 1800 calories for one month because it is hard to stay with a very restrictive eating plan for a long time. If, after one month at 1800 calories a day, you have not reached your reasonable weight goal, go back to the 1200-calorie meal plan for another month. You can repeat this cycle until you reach your reasonable weight.

SAMPLE 1200-CALORIE EATING PLAN

FOOD	PORTION	CALORIES	CHO
BREAKFAST			
240 Calories*			
33 CHO†			
Pink Grapefruit Sections	1 cup	69	18
Whole Wheat Toast	1 slice	70	13
1% Cottage Cheese	½ cup	82	3
Tea	1 cup	0	0
			Subtotal
			221 Cal
			34 CHO
LUNCH			
420 Calories			
58 CHO			
Plain Lowfat Yogurt	8 oz	144	16
Fruit Cocktail, water			
pack	½ cup	40	10
English Muffin	1	140	27
Diet Jelly	1 tbsp	6	1
Dry Roasted Peanuts	½ oz	82	3
Tea	1 cup	0	0
			Subtotal
			412 Cal
			57 CHO

*calories for a meal can be plus 25 or minus 25 calories
†carbohydrate for a meal can be plus 5 or minus 5 CHO
tr = trace

(continues on next page)

SAMPLE 1200-CALORIE EATING PLAN

FOOD	PORTION	CALORIES	CHO
DINNER			
420 Calories			
58 CHO			
Roast Chicken w/o skin	½ breast	142	0
Baked Potato w/ skin	1	220	51
Broccoli, cooked	½ cup	23	4
Tossed Salad	¾ cup	16	3
Lemon Juice & Fresh			
Pepper	1 tbsp	4	1
Diet Margarine	2 tsp	34	0
Diet Cola	12 oz	2	tr
		Subtotal	
		441 Cal	
		59 CHO	
SNACK—Evening			
120 Calories			
17 CHO			
Sliced Apple w/o Skin	1 cup	62	16
Cheddar Cheese	½ oz	57	tr
		Subtotal	
		119 Cal	
		16 CHO	
		Daily total	
1200 Calories		1193 Cal	
165 CHO		166 CHO	

1200-CALORIE EATING PLAN WORKSHEET

FOOD	PORTION	CALORIES	CHO

BREAKFAST
240 Calories*
 33 CHO†

Subtotal
_____ Cal
_____ CHO

LUNCH
420 Calories
 58 CHO

Subtotal
_____ Cal
_____ CHO

*calories for a meal can be plus 25 or minus 25 calories
†carbohydrate for a meal can be plus 5 or minus 5 CHO

(continues on next page)

1200-CALORIE EATING PLAN WORKSHEET

FOOD	PORTION	CALORIES	CHO

DINNER
420 Calories
 58 CHO

		Subtotal	
		_____ Cal	
		_____ CHO	

SNACK
120 Calories
 17 CHO

		Subtotal	
		_____ Cal	
		_____ CHO	

		Daily total	
1200 Calories		_____ Cal	
165 CHO		_____ CHO	

1500-Calorie Eating Plan

A 1500-calorie eating plan is restrictive. It's best to stay at this calorie level for one month to achieve quick weight loss. Then move to 1800 or 2100 calories for one month because it is hard to stay with a restrictive eating plan for a long time. If after one month at 1800 or 2100 calories a day you have not reached your reasonable weight goal, go back to the 1500-calorie meal plan for another month. You can repeat this cycle until you reach your reasonable weight.

SAMPLE 1500-CALORIE EATING PLAN

FOOD	PORTION	CALORIES	CHO
BREAKFAST			
300 Calories*			
41 CHO†			
Pink Grapefruit Sections	1 cup	69	18
Whole Wheat Toast	1½ slices	105	20
Creamed Cottage			
Cheese	½ cup	108	3
Tea	1 cup	0	0
			Subtotal
			282 Cal
			41 CHO

*calories for a meal can be plus 25 or minus 25 calories
†carbohydrate for a meal can be plus 5 or minus 5 CHO
tr = trace

(continues on next page)

SAMPLE 1500-CALORIE EATING PLAN

FOOD	PORTION	CALORIES	CHO
LUNCH			
525 Calories			
72 CHO			
Plain Lowfat Yogurt	8 oz	144	16
Fruit Cocktail, water			
pack	1 cup	80	20
English Muffin	1	140	27
Diet Jelly	1 tbsp	6	1
Dry Roasted Peanuts	1 oz	164	6
Tea	1 cup	0	0
		Subtotal	
		534	Cal
		70	CHO

FOOD	PORTION	CALORIES	CHO
DINNER			
525 Calories			
72 CHO			
Roast Chicken w/o skin	½ breast	142	0
Baked Potato w/ skin	1	220	51
Broccoli, cooked	½ cup	23	4
Tossed Salad	¾ cup	16	3
Thousand Island			
Dressing	1 tbsp	59	2
Dried Apricots	6 halves	50	13
Club soda	1 cup	0	0
		Subtotal	
		510	Cal
		73	CHO

SAMPLE 1500-CALORIE EATING PLAN

FOOD	PORTION	CALORIES	CHO	
SNACK—Evening				
150 Calories				
21 CHO				
Apple	1	81	21	
Cheddar Cheese	½ oz	57	tr	
				Subtotal
				138 Cal
				21 CHO
				Daily total
1500 Calories				1464 Cal
206 CHO				205 CHO

1500-CALORIE EATING PLAN WORKSHEET

FOOD	PORTION	CALORIES	CHO
BREAKFAST 300 Calories* 41 CHO†			

Subtotal
_____ Cal
_____ CHO

| **LUNCH** 525 Calories 72 CHO | | | |

Subtotal
_____ Cal
_____ CHO

*calories for a meal can be plus 25 or minus 25 calories
†carbohydrate for a meal can be plus 5 or minus 5 CHO

1500-CALORIE EATING PLAN WORKSHEET

FOOD	PORTION	CALORIES	CHO
DINNER 525 Calories 72 CHO			

	Subtotal
	_____ Cal
	_____ CHO

FOOD	PORTION	CALORIES	CHO
SNACK 150 Calories 21 CHO			

	Subtotal
	_____ Cal
	_____ CHO

	Daily total
1500 Calories	_____ Cal
206 CHO	_____ CHO

1800-Calorie Eating Plan

At 1800 calories you'll see that there is more food to eat and a greater variety of foods from which to choose. The 1800-calorie level will be a weight maintenance eating plan for most women and some men.

SAMPLE 1800-CALORIE EATING PLAN

FOOD	PORTION	CALORIES	CHO
BREAKFAST			
360 Calories*			
50 CHO†			
Pink Grapefruit Sections	1 cup	69	18
Oatmeal, cooked	½ cup	73	13
1% Milk	½ cup	51	6
Whole Wheat Toast	1 slice	70	13
Cream Cheese	1 oz	99	1
Tea	1 cup	0	0

Subtotal
362 Cal
51 CHO

*calories for a meal can be plus 25 or minus 25 calories
†carbohydrate for a meal can be plus 5 or minus 5 CHO
tr = trace

SAMPLE 1800-CALORIE EATING PLAN

FOOD	PORTION	CALORIES	CHO	
LUNCH				
630 Calories				
87 CHO				
Take-out Tuna Salad	3 oz	159	8	
Rye Bread	2 slices	130	24	
Red Tomato	1	24	5	
Iceberg Lettuce	1 leaf	3	tr	
Chickpeas, canned	½ cup	143	27	
Reduced Calorie Italian				
Dressing	1 tbsp	16	1	
1% Milk	1 cup	102	12	
Raisins	2 tbsp	54	14	
				Subtotal
				631 Cal
				91 CHO
DINNER				
630 Calories				
87 CHO				
Roast Chicken w/o skin	½ breast	142	0	
	1 drumstick	76	0	
Baked Potato w/ skin	1	220	51	
Broccoli, cooked	½ cup	23	4	
Tossed Salad	¾ cup	16	3	
Thousand Island				
Dressing	1 tbsp	59	2	
Banana	1	105	27	
				Subtotal
				641 Cal
				87 CHO

(continues on next page)

SAMPLE 1800-CALORIE EATING PLAN

FOOD	PORTION	CALORIES	CHO	
SNACK—Evening				
180 Calories				
25 CHO				
Apple	1	81	21	
Camembert	1 oz	85	tr	
Melba Toast	1	20	4	
				Subtotal
				186 Cal
				25 CHO
				Daily total
1800 Calories				1820 Cal
248 CHO				254 CHO

1800-CALORIE EATING PLAN WORKSHEET

FOOD	PORTION	CALORIES	CHO

BREAKFAST
360 Calories*
 50 CHO†

Subtotal
_____ Cal
_____ CHO

LUNCH
630 Calories
 87 CHO

Subtotal
_____ Cal
_____ CHO

*calories for a meal can be plus 25 or minus 25 calories
†carbohydrate for a meal can be plus 5 or minus 5 CHO

(continues on next page)

1800-CALORIE EATING PLAN WORKSHEET

FOOD	PORTION	CALORIES	CHO
DINNER			
630 Calories			
87 CHO			

Subtotal
_____ Cal
_____ CHO

SNACK			
180 Calories			
25 CHO			

Subtotal
_____ Cal
_____ CHO

Daily total
1800 Calories _____ Cal
248 CHO _____ CHO

2100-Calorie Eating Plan

At 2100 calories, there is an even greater quantity and selection of food. The 2100-calorie level is a maintenance eating plan for many men and some women.

SAMPLE 2100-CALORIE EATING PLAN

FOOD	PORTION	CALORIES	CHO
BREAKFAST			
420 Calories*			
58 CHO†			
Pink Grapefruit Sections	1 cup	69	18
Corn Flakes	1¼ cup (1 oz)	110	24
1% Milk	½ cup	51	6
Whole Wheat Toast	1 slice	70	13
Cream Cheese	1 oz	99	1
Tea	1 cup	0	0

	Subtotal
	399 Cal
	62 CHO

*calories for a meal can be plus 25 or minus 25 calories

†carbohydrate for a meal can be plus 5 or minus 5 CHO

tr = trace

(continues on next page)

SAMPLE 2100-CALORIE EATING PLAN

FOOD	PORTION	CALORIES	CHO
LUNCH			
735 Calories			
101 CHO			
Take-out Tuna Salad	3 oz	159	8
Rye Bread	2 slices	130	24
Red Tomato	1	24	5
Iceberg Lettuce	1 leaf	3	tr
Chickpeas, canned	½ cup	143	27
Blue Cheese Dressing	1 tbsp	77	1
1% Milk	1 cup	102	12
Pear	1	98	25
Club soda	1 cup	0	0
		Subtotal	
		736 Cal	
		102 CHO	
DINNER			
735 Calories			
101 CHO			
Roast Chicken w/o skin	½ breast	142	0
	1 drumstick	76	0
Baked Potato w/ skin	1	220	51
Broccoli, cooked	½ cup	23	4
Tossed Salad	¾ cup	16	3
Thousand Island			
Dressing	1 tbsp	59	2
Dinner Roll	1	85	14
Banana	1	105	27
Tea	1 cup	0	0
		Subtotal	
		726 Cal	
		101 CHO	

SAMPLE 2100-CALORIE EATING PLAN

FOOD	PORTION	CALORIES	CHO	
SNACK—Evening				
210 Calories				
29 CHO				
Apple	1	81	21	
Camembert	1 oz	85	tr	
Melba Toast	2	40	8	
				Subtotal
				206 Cal
				29 CHO
				Daily total
2100 Calories				2067 Cal
289 CHO				294 CHO

2100-CALORIE EATING PLAN WORKSHEET

FOOD	PORTION	CALORIES	CHO

BREAKFAST
420 Calories*
 58 CHO†

Subtotal
_____ Cal
_____ CHO

LUNCH
735 Calories
101 CHO

Subtotal
_____ Cal
_____ CHO

*calories for a meal can be plus 25 or minus 25 calories
†carbohydrate for a meal can be plus 5 or minus 5 CHO

2100-CALORIE EATING PLAN WORKSHEET

FOOD	PORTION	CALORIES	CHO

DINNER
735 Calories
101 CHO

		Subtotal	
		_____ Cal	
		_____ CHO	

SNACK
210 Calories
 29 CHO

		Subtotal	
		_____ Cal	
		_____ CHO	

		Daily total	
2100 Calories		_____ Cal	
289 CHO		_____ CHO	

2400-Calorie Eating Plan

Most people with diabetes maintain their weight on fewer than 2400 calories. This calorie level is appropriate for active people. At 2400 calories, it is more practical to divide the calories and carbohydrates into three meals and two snacks.

SAMPLE 2400-CALORIE EATING PLAN

FOOD	PORTION	CALORIES	CHO
BREAKFAST			
480 Calories*			
66 CHO†			
Pink Grapefruit Sections	1 cup	69	18
Corn Flakes	1¼ cup (1 oz)	110	24
2% Milk	1 cup	121	12
Whole Wheat Toast	1 slice	70	13
Cream Cheese	1 oz	99	1
Tea	1 cup	0	0

Subtotal	
469	Cal
68	CHO

*calories for a meal can be plus 25 or minus 25 calories
†carbohydrate for a meal can be plus 5 or minus 5 CHO
tr = trace

SAMPLE 2400-CALORIE EATING PLAN

FOOD	PORTION	CALORIES	CHO
LUNCH			
720 Calories			
99 CHO			
Take-out Tuna Salad	3 oz	159	8
Rye Bread	2 slices	130	24
Iceberg Lettuce	1 leaf	3	tr
Celery Stalk, raw	2	12	2
Chickpeas, canned	½ cup	143	27
Blue Cheese Dressing	1 tbsp	77	1
1% Milk	1 cup	102	12
Pear	1	98	25
			Subtotal
			724 Cal
			99 CHO
DINNER			
720 Calories			
99 CHO			
Roast Chicken w/o skin	½ breast	142	0
	1 drumstick	76	0
Baked Potato w/ skin	1	220	51
Broccoli, cooked	1 cup	46	8
Tossed Salad	¾ cup	16	3
Thousand Island			
Dressing	1 tbsp	59	2
Dinner Roll	1	85	14
Peach Halves, juice pack	2	76	20
Club Soda	12 oz	0	0
			Subtotal
			720 Cal
			98 CHO

(continues on next page)

SAMPLE 2400-CALORIE EATING PLAN

FOOD	PORTION	CALORIES	CHO
SNACK—Midmorning			
240 Calories			
33 CHO			
Toasted Bagel	1	200	38
Diet Margarine	2 tsp	34	0
			Subtotal
			234 Cal
			38 CHO

FOOD	PORTION	CALORIES	CHO
SNACK—Evening			
240 Calories			
33 CHO			
Apple	1	81	21
Camembert	1 oz	85	tr
Melba Toast	3	60	12
			Subtotal
			226 Cal
			33 CHO

FOOD	PORTION	CALORIES	CHO
			Daily total
2400 Calories			2373 Cal
330 CHO			336 CHO

2400-CALORIE EATING PLAN WORKSHEET

FOOD	PORTION	CALORIES	CHO

BREAKFAST
480 Calories*
 66 CHO†

Subtotal		
_____	Cal	
_____	CHO	

LUNCH
720 Calories
 99 CHO

Subtotal		
_____	Cal	
_____	CHO	

*calories for a meal can be plus 25 or minus 25 calories
†carbohydrate for a meal can be plus 5 or minus 5 CHO

(continues on next page)

2400-CALORIE EATING PLAN WORKSHEET

FOOD	PORTION	CALORIES	CHO

DINNER
720 Calories
 99 CHO

Subtotal
_____ Cal
_____ CHO

SNACK
240 Calories
 33 CHO

Subtotal
_____ Cal
_____ CHO

2400-CALORIE EATING PLAN WORKSHEET

FOOD	PORTION	CALORIES	CHO

SNACK
240 Calories
 33 CHO

Subtotal
_____ Cal
_____ CHO

Daily total
2400 Calories _____ Cal
 330 CHO _____ CHO

2700-Calorie Eating Plan

Most people with Type II diabetes maintain their weight on fewer than 2700 calories. This calorie level is appropriate for very active people. At 2700 calories it is more practical to divide the calories and carbohydrates into three meals and three snacks.

SAMPLE 2700-CALORIE EATING PLAN

FOOD	PORTION	CALORIES	CHO
BREAKFAST			
540 Calories*			
74 CHO†			
Pink Grapefruit Sections	1 cup	69	18
Bran Flakes	¾ cup	90	22
	(1 oz)		
2% Milk	1 cup	121	12
Whole Wheat Toast	2 slices	140	26
Cream Cheese	1 oz	99	1

Subtotal
519 Cal
79 CHO

*calories for a meal can be plus 25 or minus 25 calories
†carbohydrate for a meal can be plus 5 or minus 5 CHO
tr = trace

SAMPLE 2700-CALORIE EATING PLAN

FOOD	PORTION	CALORIES	CHO	
LUNCH				
675 Calories				
93 CHO				
Take-out Tuna Salad	3 oz	159	8	
Rye Bread	2 slices	130	24	
Iceberg Lettuce	1 leaf	3	tr	
Chickpeas, canned	½ cup	143	27	
Blue Cheese Dressing	1 tbsp	77	1	
1% Milk	1 cup	102	12	
Tangerine	2	74	18	
				Subtotal
				688 Cal
				90 CHO
DINNER				
675 Calories				
93 CHO				
Roast Chicken w/o skin	½ breast	142	0	
	1 drumstick	76	0	
Baked Potato w/ skin	1	220	51	
Broccoli, cooked	½ cup	23	4	
Tossed Salad	¾ cup	16	3	
Thousand Island				
Dressing	1 tbsp	59	2	
Dinner Roll	1	85	14	
Peach Halves, juice pack	2	76	20	
Club Soda	1 cup	0	0	
				Subtotal
				697 Cal
				94 CHO

(continues on next page)

SAMPLE 2700-CALORIE EATING PLAN

FOOD	PORTION	CALORIES	CHO
SNACK—Midmorning			
270 Calories			
37 CHO			
Toasted Bagel	1	200	38
Mozzarella, part skim	1 oz	72	1
		Subtotal	
		272 Cal	
		39 CHO	
SNACK—Midafternoon			
270 Calories			
37 CHO			
Lowfat Plain Yogurt	8 oz	144	16
Toasted Wheat Germ	2 tbsp	54	7
Purple Plums, juice pack	½ cup	73	19
		Subtotal	
		271 Cal	
		42 CHO	
SNACK—Evening			
270 Calories			
37 CHO			
Apple	1	81	21
Colby Cheese	1 oz	112	1
Melba Toast	3	60	12
		Subtotal	
		253 Cal	
		34 CHO	
		Daily total	
2700 Calories		2700 Cal	
371 CHO		378 CHO	

2700-CALORIE EATING PLAN WORKSHEET

FOOD	PORTION	CALORIES	CHO
BREAKFAST 540 Calories* 74 CHO†			

Subtotal
_____ Cal
_____ CHO

*calories for a meal can be plus 25 or minus 25 calories
†carbohydrate for a meal can be plus 5 or minus 5 CHO

(continues on next page)

2700-CALORIE EATING PLAN WORKSHEET

FOOD	PORTION	CALORIES	CHO
LUNCH 675 Calories 93 CHO			

Subtotal
_____ Cal
_____ CHO

| **DINNER**
675 Calories
  93 CHO | | | |

Subtotal
_____ Cal
_____ CHO

| **SNACK**
270 Calories
  37 CHO | | | |

Subtotal
_____ Cal
_____ CHO

2700-CALORIE EATING PLAN WORKSHEET

FOOD	PORTION	CALORIES	CHO

SNACK
270 Calories
37 CHO

	Subtotal	
	Cal	
	CHO	

SNACK
270 Calories
37 CHO

	Subtotal	
	Cal	
	CHO	

	Daily total	
2700 Calories	Cal	
371 CHO	CHO	

5

USING THE DIABETES COUNTER

The Diabetes Counter was written for you to use as a reference while following your diabetic meal plan. All the information you need is here in one handy guide.

The Diabetes Counter lists the calories, carbohydrate and fat content of 3000 commonly eaten foods. In addition *The Diabetes Counter* marks with an asterisk which of these foods are high in sugar and should be eaten only on occasion and even then only in small amounts. Fat values are given to alert you to those foods high in fat. When you choose these, keep portions small and use them less frequently.

Before *The Diabetes Counter* it was harder to work out a meal plan. Now everything you need to know is at your fingertips—the calorie and carbohydrate value of most foods eaten, a guide to sugar in food and a guide to foods high in fat—so you can plan healthy lowfat meals.

The foods are listed alphabetically from A to Z. Within each category you will often find subcategories. For example, the category CARROTS, listed on page 116, is broken down into the subcategories "canned," "fresh," "frozen" and "juice." Many categories have "take-out" and "home recipe" subcategories to help you estimate the nutritional value of items you may make at home or order when eating out.

Apparent inconsistencies in nutrient values may result from rounding off numbers, and because values may have been obtained from various sources and/or samples of the same food. Nutrient variations in foods occur because of differences in soil content, season, processing and method of preparation, among other factors.

DEFINITIONS

as prep (as prepared): refers to food that has been prepared according to package directions

cooked: refers to food cooked without the addition of fat (oil, butter, margarine, etc.); steaming, broiling and dry roasting are examples of this type of preparation

home recipe: describes homemade dishes; those included can be used as a guide to the carbohydrate, fat, sugar and calorie values of similar products

take-out: describes products you buy ready-to-eat or restaurant menu items

trace (tr): values used when a food contains less than one calorie, less than one gram of carbohydrate or less than one gram of fat

0" trim: all visible fat removed from outer edge of meat

¼" trim: visible fat trimmed to within ¼ inch

ABBREVIATIONS

*	= high in added sugar	qt	= quart
diam	= diameter	reg	= regular
frzn	= frozen	sm	= small
g	= gram	sq	= square
lb	= pound	tbsp	= tablespoon
lg	= large	tr	= trace
med	= medium	tsp	= teaspoon
oz	= ounce	w/	= with
pkg	= package	w/o	= without
prep	= prepared	"	= inch

EQUIVALENT MEASURES

1 tablespoon = 3 teaspoons
4 tablespoons = ¼ cup
8 tablespoons = ½ cup
12 tablespoons = ¾ cup
16 tablespoons = 1 cup
28 grams   = 1 ounce

DRY MEASUREMENTS	LIQUID MEASUREMENTS
16 ounces = 1 pound	2 tablespoons = 1 ounce
12 ounces = ¾ pound	¼ cup = 2 ounces
8 ounces = ½ pound	½ cup = 4 ounces
4 ounces = ¼ pound	¾ cup = 6 ounces
	1 cup = 8 ounces
	2 cups = 16 ounces
	2 cups = 1 pint
	4 cups = 32 ounces
	4 cups = 1 quart

ALL CHO (CARBOHYDRATE) AND FAT VALUES ARE GIVEN IN GRAMS.

*INDICATES FOODS HIGH IN ADDED SUGAR THAT SHOULD BE EATEN ONLY OCCASIONALLY AND, EVEN THEN, IN SMALL AMOUNTS.

THE DIABETES
CARBOHYDRATE AND CALORIE
COUNTER

FOOD	PORTION	CALORIES	CHO	FAT
ABALONE				
FRESH				
fried	3 oz	161	9	6
raw	3 oz	89	5	1
ACEROLA				
acerola	1 fruit	2	tr	tr
JUICE				
acerola	1 cup	51	12	1
ADZUKI BEANS				
CANNED				
*sweetened	1 cup	702	163	tr
DRIED				
cooked	1 cup	294	57	tr
raw	1 cup	649	124	1
READY-TO-USE				
*yokan; sliced	3¼" slice	112	26	tr
AKEE				
fresh	3½ oz	223	5	20
ALFALFA				
sprouts	1 cup	40	1	tr
sprouts	1 tbsp	1	tr	tr
ALLSPICE				
ground	1 tsp	5	1	tr

FOOD	PORTION	CALORIES	CHO	FAT
ALMONDS				
almond butter w/o salt	1 tbsp	101	3	10
*almond butter, honey & cinnamon	1 tbsp	96	4	8
almond meal	1 oz	116	8	5
almond paste	1 oz	127	12	8
dried, blanched	1 oz	166	5	15
dried, unblanched	1 oz	167	6	15
dry roasted, unblanched	1 oz	167	7	15
dry roasted, unblanched, salted	1 oz	167	7	15
oil roasted, blanched	1 oz	174	5	16
oil roasted, blanched, salted	1 oz	174	5	16
oil roasted, unblanched	1 oz	176	5	16
oil roasted, unblanched, salted	1 oz	176	5	16
toasted, unblanched	1 oz	167	7	14
AMARANTH				
cooked	½ cup	59	3	tr
uncooked	½ cup	366	65	6
ANCHOVY				
CANNED				
in oil	5	42	0	2
in oil	1 can (1.6 oz)	95	0	4

FOOD	PORTION	CALORIES	CHO	FAT
FRESH				
raw	3 oz	62	0	4
ANGLERFISH				
raw	3½ oz	72	0	1
ANISE				
seed	1 tsp	7	1	tr
APPLE				
CANNED				
*applesauce, sweetened	½ cup	97	25	tr
applesauce, unsweetened	½ cup	53	14	tr
*sliced, sweetened	1 cup	136	34	1
DRIED				
*cooked w/ sugar	½ cup	116	29	tr
cooked w/o sugar	½ cup	72	20	tr
rings	10	155	42	tr
FRESH				
apple	1	81	21	tr
w/o skin; sliced	1 cup	62	16	tr
w/o skin; sliced & microwaved	1 cup	96	25	tr
w/o skin; sliced & cooked	1 cup	91	23	tr
FROZEN				
sliced, w/o sugar	½ cup	41	11	tr
JUICE				
apple	1 cup	116	29	tr

FOOD	PORTION	CALORIES	CHO	FAT
frzn; as prep	1 cup	111	28	tr
frzn; not prep	6 oz	349	87	1

APRICOTS

CANNED

*heavy syrup w/ skin	3 halves	70	18	tr
juice pack w/ skin	3 halves	40	10	tr
*light syrup w/ skin	3 halves	54	14	tr
water pack w/ skin	3 halves	22	5	tr
water pack w/o skin	4 halves	20	5	tr

DRIED

halves	10	83	22	tr
halves; cooked w/o sugar	½ cup	106	27	tr

FRESH

apricots	3	51	12	tr

FROZEN

*sweetened	½ cup	119	30	tr

JUICE

nectar	1 cup	141	36	tr

ARROWHEAD

fresh; boiled	1 med (⅓ oz)	9	2	tr

ARROWROOT

flour	1 cup	457	113	tr

ARTICHOKE

FRESH

boiled	1 med	53	12	tr

FOOD	PORTION	CALORIES	CHO	FAT
hearts; cooked	½ cup	37	9	tr
Jerusalem, raw; sliced	½ cup	57	13	tr
FROZEN				
cooked	1 pkg (9 oz)	108	22	1

ASPARAGUS

CANNED				
spears	½ cup	24	3	1
FRESH				
cooked	½ cup	22	4	tr
cooked	4 spears	15	3	tr
raw	½ cup	15	2	tr
FROZEN				
cooked	4 spears	17	3	tr
cooked	1 pkg (10 oz)	82	14	1

AVOCADO

FRESH				
avocado	1	324	15	31
puree	1 cup	370	17	35

BACON

breakfast strips, beef; cooked	3 strips (34 g)	153	tr	12
cooked	3 strips	109	tr	9
grilled	2 slices (1.7 oz)	86	1	4

FOOD	PORTION	CALORIES	CHO	FAT

BACON SUBSTITUTES

bacon substitute	1 strip	25	1	2

BAGEL

egg	1 (3½" diam)	200	38	2
plain	1 (3½" diam)	200	38	2

BAKING POWDER

baking powder	1 tsp	5	1	0
low sodium	1 tsp	5	1	0

BALSAM PEAR

leafy tips, raw	½ cup	7	1	tr
leafy tips; cooked	½ cup	10	2	tr
pods; cooked	½ cup	12	3	tr

BAMBOO SHOOTS

CANNED				
sliced	1 cup	25	4	1
FRESH				
cooked	½ cup	15	2	tr
raw	½ cup	21	1	tr

BANANA

DRIED				
powder	1 tbsp	21	5	tr
FRESH				
banana	1	105	27	tr

FOOD	PORTION	CALORIES	CHO	FAT
BARLEY				
pearled; cooked	½ cup	97	30	tr
pearled, uncooked	½ cup	352	78	1
BASIL				
ground	1 tsp	4	1	tr
BASS				
FRESH				
freshwater, raw	3 oz	97	0	3
sea, raw	3 oz	82	0	2
sea; cooked	3 oz	105	0	2
striped, raw	3 oz	82	0	2
BAY LEAF				
crumbled	1 tsp	2	tr	tr
BEANS				
CANNED				
baked beans, plain	½ cup	118	26	1
baked beans, vegetarian	½ cup	118	26	1
baked beans w/ beef	½ cup	161	22	5
baked beans w/ franks	½ cup	182	20	8
baked beans w/ pork	½ cup	133	25	2
baked beans w/ pork & sweet sauce	½ cup	140	26	2
baked beans w/ pork & tomato sauce	½ cup	123	24	1

FOOD	PORTION	CALORIES	CHO	FAT
HOME RECIPE				
baked beans	½ cup	190	27	6
BEECHNUTS				
dried	1 oz	164	10	14
BEEF				
FRESH				
bottom round, lean & fat, trim 0", Choice; roasted	3 oz	172	0	8
bottom round, lean & fat, trim 0", Select; braised	3 oz	171	0	6
bottom round, lean & fat, trim 0", Select; roasted	3 oz	150	0	24
bottom round, lean & fat, trim 0"; braised	3 oz	193	0	26
bottom round, lean & fat, trim ¼", Choice; braised	3 oz	241	0	15
bottom round, lean & fat, trim ¼", Choice; roasted	3 oz	221	0	14
bottom round, lean & fat, trim ¼", Select; braised	3 oz	220	0	13
bottom round, lean & fat, trim ¼", Select; roasted	3 oz	199	0	11
brisket, flat half, lean & fat, trim 0"; braised	3 oz	183	0	8
brisket, flat half, lean & fat, trim ¼"; braised	3 oz	309	0	24
brisket, point half, lean & fat, trim 0"; braised	3 oz	304	0	24

FOOD	PORTION	CALORIES	CHO	FAT
brisket, point half, lean & fat, trim ¼"; braised	3 oz	343	0	29
brisket, whole, lean & fat, trim 0"; braised	3 oz	247	0	17
brisket, whole, lean & fat, trim ¼", raw	1 oz	88	0	8
brisket, whole, lean & fat, trim ¼"; braised	3 oz	327	0	27
chuck arm pot roast, lean & fat, trim 0"; braised	3 oz	238	0	14
chuck arm pot roast, lean & fat, trim ¼"; braised	3 oz	282	0	20
chuck blade roast, lean & fat, trim 0"; braised	3 oz	284	0	21
chuck blade roast, lean & fat, trim ¼ "; braised	3 oz	293	0	22
corned beef brisket, raw	4 oz	56	tr	4
corned beef brisket; cooked	3 oz	213	tr	16
eye of round, lean & fat, trim 0", Choice; roasted	3 oz	153	0	5
eye of round, lean & fat, trim 0", Select; roasted	3 oz	137	0	4
eye of round, lean & fat, trim ¼", Choice; roasted	3 oz	205	0	12
eye of round, lean & fat, trim ¼"; raw	1 oz	60	0	4
eye of round, lean & fat, trim ¼", Select; roasted	3 oz	184	0	10

FOOD	PORTION	CALORIES	CHO	FAT
flank, lean & fat, trim 0"; braised	3 oz	224	0	14
flank, lean & fat, trim 0"; broiled	3 oz	192	0	11
ground lean; broiled well done	3 oz	238	0	15
ground regular, raw	4 oz	351	0	30
ground regular; broiled medium	3 oz	246	0	18
ground regular; broiled well done	3 oz	248	0	17
ground, extra lean, raw	4 oz	265	0	19
ground, extra lean; broiled medium	3 oz	217	0	14
ground, extra lean; broiled well done	3 oz	225	0	14
ground, extra lean; fried medium	3 oz	216	0	14
ground, extra lean; fried well done	3 oz	224	0	14
ground, lean, raw	4 oz	298	0	23
ground, lean; broiled medium	3 oz	231	0	16
porterhouse steak, lean only, trim ¼", Choice; broiled	3 oz	185	0	9
porterhouse steak, lean & fat, trim ¼", Choice; broiled	3 oz	260	0	19

FOOD	PORTION	CALORIES	CHO	FAT
rib eye small end, lean & fat, trim 0", Choice; broiled	3 oz	261	0	19
rib large end, lean & fat, trim 0"; roasted	3 oz	300	0	24
rib large end, lean & fat, trim ¼"; broiled	3 oz	295	0	24
rib large end, lean & fat, trim ¼"; roasted	3 oz	310	0	25
rib small end, lean & fat, trim 0"; broiled	3 oz	252	0	18
rib small end, lean & fat, trim ¼"; broiled	3 oz	285	0	22
rib small end, lean & fat, trim ¼"; roasted	3 oz	295	0	24
rib whole, lean & fat, trim ¼", Choice; broiled	3 oz	306	0	25
rib whole, lean & fat, trim ¼", Choice; roasted	3 oz	320	0	27
rib whole, lean & fat, trim ¼", Prime; roasted	3 oz	348	0	30
rib whole, lean & fat, trim ¼", Select; broiled	3 oz	274	0	21
rib whole, lean & fat, trim ¼", Select; roasted	3 oz	286	0	23
shank crosscut, lean & fat, trim ¼", Choice; simmered	3 oz	224	0	12
short loin top loin, lean & fat, trim 0", Choice; broiled	3 oz	193	0	10
short loin top loin, lean & fat, trim 0", Choice; broiled	1 steak (5.4 oz)	353	0	19

FOOD	PORTION	CALORIES	CHO	FAT
short loin top loin, lean & fat, trim 0", Select; broiled	1 steak (5.4 oz)	309	0	14
short loin top loin, lean & fat, trim ¼", Choice, raw	1 steak (8.3 oz)	611	0	47
short loin top loin, lean & fat, trim ¼", Choice; broiled	3 oz	253	0	18
short loin top loin, lean & fat, trim ¼", Choice; broiled	1 steak (6.3 oz)	536	0	38
short loin top loin, lean & fat, trim ¼", Select; broiled	1 steak (6.3 oz)	473	0	31
short loin top loin, lean & fat, trim ¼", Prime, broiled	1 steak (6.3 oz)	582	0	43
short loin top loin, lean only, trim 0", Choice; broiled	1 steak (5.2 oz)	311	0	14
short loin top loin, lean only, trim ¼", Choice; broiled	1 steak (5.2 oz)	314	0	15
shortribs, lean & fat, Choice; braised	3 oz	400	0	36
t-bone steak, lean & fat, trim ¼", Choice; broiled	3 oz	253	0	18
t-bone steak, lean only, trim ¼", Choice; broiled	3 oz	182	0	9
tenderloin, lean & fat, trim ¼", Choice; broiled	3 oz	259	0	19
tenderloin, lean & fat, trim ¼", Choice; roasted	3 oz	288	0	22
tenderloin, lean & fat, trim ¼", Prime; broiled	3 oz	270	0	20

FOOD	PORTION	CALORIES	CHO	FAT
tenderloin, lean & fat, trim ¼", Select; roasted	3 oz	275	0	21
tenderloin, lean & fat, trim ¼", raw	1 oz	80	0	7
tenderloin, lean & fat, trim 0", Choice; broiled	3 oz	208	0	12
tenderloin, lean & fat, trim 0", Select; broiled	3 oz	194	0	11
tenderloin, lean only, trim 0", Select; broiled	3 oz	170	0	7
tenderloin, lean only, trim ¼", Choice; broiled	3 oz	188	0	10
tenderloin, lean only, trim ¼", Select; broiled	3 oz	169	0	7
tip round, lean & fat, trim ¼", Choice; roasted	3 oz	210	0	13
tip round, lean & fat, trim ¼", Prime; roasted	3 oz	233	0	15
tip round, lean & fat, trim ¼", Select; roasted	3 oz	191	0	10
tip round, lean & fat, trim 0", Choice; roasted	3 oz	170	0	8
tip round, lean & fat, trim 0", Select; roasted	3 oz	158	0	6
top round, lean & fat, trim ¼", Choice; braised	3 oz	221	0	11
top round, lean & fat, trim ¼", Choice; broiled	3 oz	190	0	9
top round, lean & fat, trim ¼", Choice; fried	3 oz	235	0	13

FOOD	PORTION	CALORIES	CHO	FAT
top round, lean & fat, trim ¼", Prime; broiled	3 oz	195	0	9
top round, lean & fat, trim ¼", Select; braised	3 oz	199	0	8
top round, lean & fat, trim ¼", Select; broiled	3 oz	175	0	7
top round, lean & fat, trim ¼", raw	1 oz	50	0	3
top round, lean & fat, trim 0", Choice: braised	3 oz	184	0	6
top round, lean & fat, trim 0", Select; braised	3 oz	170	0	5
top sirloin, lean & fat, trim 0", Choice; broiled	3 oz	194	0	10
top sirloin, lean & fat, trim 0", Select; broiled	3 oz	166	0	6
top sirloin, lean & fat, trim ¼", Choice; broiled	3 oz	228	0	14
top sirloin, lean & fat, trim ¼", Choice; fried	3 oz	277	0	19
top sirloin, lean & fat, trim ¼", Select; broiled	3 oz	208	0	12
tripe, raw	4 oz	111	0	4
FROZEN patties, raw	4 oz	319	0	26
patties; broiled medium	3 oz	240	0	17

FOOD	PORTION	CALORIES	CHO	FAT
BEEF DISHES				
HOME RECIPE				
stew w/ vegetables	1 cup	220	15	11
TAKE-OUT				
roast beef sandwich w/ cheese	1	402	27	18
roast beef sandwich, plain	1	346	33	14
roast beef submarine sandwich w/ tomato, lettuce, mayonnaise	1	411	44	13
steak sandwich w/ tomato, lettuce, salt, mayonnaise	1	459	52	14
BEEFALO				
raw	1 oz	41	0	1
roasted	3 oz	160	0	5
BEER AND ALE				
beer, light	12 oz can	100	5	0
beer, regular	12 oz can	146	13	0
BEETS				
CANNED				
*Harvard	½ cup	89	22	tr
pickled	½ cup	75	19	tr
sliced	½ cup	27	6	tr
FRESH				
beet greens, raw; chopped	½ cup	4	1	tr
beet greens, raw	½ cup	4	1	tr

FOOD	PORTION	CALORIES	CHO	FAT
beet greens; cooked	½ cup	20	4	tr
cooked	½ cup	26	6	tr
raw; sliced	½ cup	30	7	tr
JUICE				
beet juice	3½ oz	36	8	0

BISCUIT

biscuit	1 (1 oz)	100	13	5
MIX				
biscuit	1 (1 oz)	95	14	3
REFRIGERATED				
biscuit	1 (¾ oz)	65	10	2
TAKE-OUT				
plain	1	276	13	34
w/ egg	1	315	24	20
w/ egg & bacon	1	457	29	31
w/ egg & sausage	1	582	41	39
w/ egg & steak	1	474	37	28
w/ egg, cheese & bacon	1	477	33	31
w/ ham	1	387	44	18
w/ sausage	1	485	40	32
w/ steak	1	456	44	26

BISON

raw	1 oz	31	0	1
roasted	3 oz	122	0	2

FOOD	PORTION	CALORIES	CHO	FAT

BLACK BEANS

DRIED

| cooked | 1 cup | 227 | 41 | 1 |
| raw | 1 cup | 661 | 121 | 3 |

BLACKBERRIES

CANNED

| *in heavy syrup | ½ cup | 118 | 30 | tr |

FRESH

| blackberries | ½ cup | 37 | 9 | tr |

FROZEN

| unsweetened | 1 cup | 97 | 24 | 1 |

BLUEBERRIES

CANNED

| *in heavy syrup | 1 cup | 225 | 56 | 1 |

FRESH

| blueberries | 1 cup | 82 | 20 | 1 |

FROZEN

| unsweetened | 1 cup | 78 | 19 | 1 |

BLUEFISH

FRESH

| raw | 3 oz | 105 | 0 | 4 |

BORAGE

FRESH

| cooked; chopped | 3½ oz | 25 | 4 | 1 |
| raw; chopped | ½ cup | 9 | 1 | tr |

FOOD	PORTION	CALORIES	CHO	FAT

BOYSENBERRIES

CANNED
*in heavy syrup

	1 cup	226	57	tr

FROZEN
unsweetened

	1 cup	66	16	tr

BRAINS

beef; pan-fried	3 oz	167	0	13
beef; simmered	3 oz	136	0	11
lamb; braised	3 oz	124	0	9
lamb; fried	3 oz	232	0	19
pork, raw	3 oz	108	0	8
pork; braised	3 oz	117	0	8
veal; braised	3 oz	115	0	8
veal; fried	3 oz	181	0	14

BRAN

corn; cooked	⅓ cup	56	21	tr
oat, dry	½ cup	116	31	3
oat; cooked	½ cup	44	13	tr
rice, dry	⅓ cup	88	14	6
wheat, dry	½ cup	65	19	1

BRAZIL NUTS

dried, unblanched	1 oz	186	4	19

FOOD	PORTION	CALORIES	CHO	FAT
BREAD				
CANNED				
Boston brown	1 slice	95	21	1
HOME RECIPE				
hush puppies	5 (2.7 oz)	256	35	12
READY-TO-EAT				
cracked wheat	1 slice	65	12	1
cracked wheat; toasted	1 slice	65	12	1
French	1 loaf (1 lb)	454	230	18
French	1 slice (1.2 oz)	100	18	1
Italian	1 loaf (1 lb)	454	256	4
Italian	1 slice (1 oz)	85	17	tr
oatmeal	1 slice	65	12	1
pita	1 (2 oz)	165	33	1
pumpernickel	1 slice	80	16	1
raisin	1 slice	65	13	1
rye	1 slice	65	12	1
Vienna	1 slice (.9 oz)	70	13	1
wheat	1 slice	65	12	1
white	1 slice	65	12	1
white; cubed	1 cup	80	15	1
whole wheat	1 slice	70	13	1
BREADCRUMBS				
dry	1 cup	390	73	5
fresh	1 cup	120	22	2

FOOD	PORTION	CALORIES	CHO	FAT

BREADFRUIT

FOOD	PORTION	CALORIES	CHO	FAT
fresh	¼ small	99	26	tr
seeds, raw	1 oz	54	8	9
seeds, roasted	1 oz	59	11	tr
seeds, cooked	1 oz	48	9	•

BREADNUTTREE SEEDS

FOOD	PORTION	CALORIES	CHO	FAT
dried	1 oz	104	23	b

BREAKFAST DRINKS

FOOD	PORTION	CALORIES	CHO	FAT
*orange drink powder; as prep w/ water	6 oz	86	22	0
*orange drink, powder	3 rounded tsp	93	24	0

BROAD BEANS

FOOD	PORTION	CALORIES	CHO	FAT
CANNED				
broad beans	1 cup	183	32	
DRIED				
cooked	1 cup	186	33	1
raw	1 cup	511	87	2
FRESH				
cooked	3½ oz	56	10	tr

BROCCOLI

FOOD	PORTION	CALORIES	CHO	FAT
FRESH				
chopped, cooked	½ cup	23	4	tr
raw, chopped	½ cup	12	2	tr
FROZEN				
chopped, cooked	½ cup	25	5	tr

FOOD	PORTION	CALORIES	CHO	FAT
spears; cooked	10 oz pkg	69	13	tr
spears; cooked	½ cup	25	5	tr

BROWNIE

HOME RECIPE
| *w/ nuts | 1 (.8 oz) | 95 | 11 | 6 |

READY-TO-EAT
| *w/ nuts | 1 (1 oz) | 100 | 16 | 4 |
| *w/o nuts | 1 (2 oz) | 243 | 39 | 10 |

BRUSSELS SPROUTS

FRESH
cooked	½ cup	30	7	tr
cooked	1 sprout	8	2	tr
raw	½ cup	19	4	tr
raw	1 sprout	8	2	tr

FROZEN
| cooked | ½ cup | 33 | 6 | tr |

BUCKWHEAT

flour, whole groat	1 cup	402	85	4
groats, roasted: uncooked	½ cup	283	61	2
groats, roasted; cooked	½ cup	91	20	tr

BUFFALO

| water, raw | 1 oz | 28 | 0 | tr |
| water; roasted | 3 oz | 111 | 0 | 2 |

FOOD	PORTION	CALORIES	CHO	FAT
BULGUR				
cooked	½ cup	76	17	tr
uncooked	½ cup	239	53	tr
BURBOT (FISH)				
FRESH				
raw	3 oz	76	0	1
BURDOCK ROOT				
cooked	1 cup	110	26	tr
raw	1 cup	85	20	tr
BUTTER				
REGULAR				
butter	1 pat	36	tr	4
butter	1 stick (4 oz)	813	tr	92
butter oil	1 cup	1795	0	204
butter oil	1 tbsp	112	0	13
clarified butter	3½ oz	876	0	99
WHIPPED				
butter	1 pat	27	tr	3
butter	4 oz	542	tr	61
BUTTERBUR				
CANNED				
fuki, chopped	1 cup	3	tr	tr
FRESH				
fuki, raw	1 cup	13	3	tr

FOOD	PORTION	CALORIES	CHO	FAT
BUTTERFISH				
raw	3 oz	124	0	7
BUTTERNUTS				
dried	1 oz	174	3	16
CABBAGE				
FRESH				
Chinese, pak-choi, raw; shredded	½ cup	5	1	tr
Chinese pak-choi; shredded, cooked	½ cup	10	2	tr
Chinese, pe-tsai, raw; shredded	1 cup	12	2	tr
Chinese, pe-tsai; shredded, cooked	1 cup	16	3	tr
green, raw; shredded	½ cup	8	2	tr
green, raw; shredded	1 head (2 lbs)	215	49	2
green; shredded, cooked	½ cup	16	4	tr
red, raw; shredded	½ cup	10	2	tr
red; shredded, cooked	½ cup	16	3	tr
Savoy, raw; shredded	½ cup	10	2	tr
Savoy; shredded, cooked	½ cup	18	4	tr
HOME RECIPE				
coleslaw	½ cup	42	7	2
coleslaw w/ dressing	¾ cup	147	13	11

FOOD	PORTION	CALORIES	CHO	FAT
CAKE				
*carrot w/ cream cheese icing	1 cake 10" diam	6175	775	328
*carrot w/ cream cheese icing	1/16 of cake	385	48	21
*fruitcake, dark	1 cake 7½" × 2¼"	5185	738	228
*fruitcake, dark	⅔ slice	165	25	7
*pound cake	1 loaf 8½" × 3½"	1935	265	94
*pound cake	1 slice (1 oz)	120	15	5
*sheet cake w/ white frosting	⅑ of cake	445	77	14
*sheet cake w/ white frosting	1 cake 9" sq	4020	694	129
*sheet cake w/o frosting	1 cake 9" sq	2830	434	108
*sheet cake w/o frosting	⅑ of cake	315	48	12
MIX				
*angelfood	1 cake 9¾" diam	1510	342	2
*angelfood	1/12 of cake	125	29	tr
*crumb coffeecake	1 cake 7¾" × 5⅝"	1385	225	41
*crumb coffeecake	⅙ of cake	230	38	7
*devil's food cupcake w/ chocolate frosting	1	120	20	4
*devil's food w/ chocolate frosting	1 cake 9" diam	3755	645	136
*devil's food w/ chocolate frosting	1/16 of cake	235	40	8

FOOD	PORTION	CALORIES	CHO	FAT
*gingerbread	1 cake 8″ sq	1575	291	39
*gingerbread	1/9 of cake	175	32	4
*yellow w/ chocolate frosting; as prep	1 cake 9″ diam	3735	638	125
*yellow w/ chocolate frosting; as prep	1/16 of cake	235	40	8
READY-TO-USE				
*cheesecake	1 cake 9″ diam	3350	317	213
*cheesecake	1/12 of cake	280	26	18
*pound cake	1 cake (8½″ × 3½″ × 3″)	1935	257	94
*pound cake	1 slice (1 oz)	110	15	12
*white w/ white frosting	1 cake 9″ diam	4170	670	148
*white w/ white frosting	1/16 of cake	260	42	9
*yellow w/ chocolate frosting	1 cake 9″ diam	3895	620	175
*yellow w/ chocolate frosting	1/16 of cake	245	39	11
SNACK				
*devil's food w/ creme filling	1 (1 oz)	105	17	4
*sponge w/ creme filling	1 (1.5 oz)	155	27	5
*toaster pastries	1 (1.9 oz)	210	38	6

CANADIAN BACON

FOOD	PORTION	CALORIES	CHO	FAT
unheated	2 slices (1.9 oz)	89	1	4

FOOD	PORTION	CALORIES	CHO	FAT

CANDY

FOOD	PORTION	CALORIES	CHO	FAT
*candy corn	1 oz	105	27	0
*caramels, chocolate	1 oz	115	22	3
*caramels, plain	1 oz	115	22	3
*chocolate	1 oz	145	16	9
*chocolate crisp	1 oz	140	18	7
*chocolate w/ almonds	1 oz	150	15	10
*chocolate w/ peanuts	1 oz	155	13	11
*dark chocolate	1 oz	150	16	10
*fudge, chocolate	1 oz	115	21	3
*fudge, vanilla	1 oz	115	21	3
*gum drops	1 oz	100	25	tr
*hard candy	1 oz	110	28	0
*jelly beans	1 oz	105	26	tr
*marshmallow	1 oz	90	23	0
*marzipan	3½ oz	497	57	25
*mint fondant	1 oz	105	27	0
*nougat nut cream	3½ oz	342	58	31

CANTALOUP

FOOD	PORTION	CALORIES	CHO	FAT
cubed	1 cup	57	13	tr
fresh	½	94	22	1

CARAMBOLA

FOOD	PORTION	CALORIES	CHO	FAT
fresh	1	42	10	tr

FOOD	PORTION	CALORIES	CHO	FAT

CARAWAY

| seed | 1 tsp | 7 | 1 | tr |

CARDAMON

| ground | 1 tsp | 6 | 1 | tr |

CARDOON

FRESH

| cooked | 3½ oz | 22 | 5 | tr |
| raw; shredded | ½ cup | 36 | 4 | tr |

CARIBOU

| raw | 1 oz | 36 | 0 | 1 |
| roasted | 3 oz | 142 | 0 | 4 |

CARISSA

| fresh | 1 | 12 | 3 | tr |

CAROB

*carob mix	3 tsp	45	11	0
*carob mix: as prep w/ whole milk	9 oz	195	23	8
flour	1 cup	185	92	1
flour	1 tbsp	14	7	tr

CARP

FRESH

| cooked | 3 oz | 138 | 0 | 6 |

FOOD	PORTION	CALORIES	CHO	FAT
cooked	1 fillet (6 oz)	276	0	12
raw	3 oz	108	0	5

CARROTS

CANNED

slices	½ cup	17	4	tr

FRESH

raw	1 (2.5 oz)	31	7	tr
raw; shredded	½ cup	24	6	tr
slices; cooked	½ cup	35	8	tr

FROZEN

slices; cooked	½ cup	26	6	tr

JUICE

canned	6 oz	73	17	tr

CASABA

cubed	1 cup	45	11	tr
fresh	⅟₁₀	43	10	tr

CASHEWS

cashew butter w/o salt	1 tbsp	94	4	8
dry roasted	1 oz	163	9	13
dry roasted, salted	1 oz	163	9	13
oil roasted	1 oz	163	8	14
oil roasted, salted	1 oz	163	8	14

FOOD	PORTION	CALORIES	CHO	FAT
CASSAVA				
FRESH				
raw	3½ oz	120	27	tr
CATFISH				
channel, raw	3 oz	99	0	4
channel; breaded & fried	3 oz	194	7	11
CATSUP				
catsup	1 tbsp	15	4	tr
CAULIFLOWER				
FRESH				
cooked	½ cup	15	3	tr
raw	½ cup	12	2	tr
FROZEN				
cooked	½ cup	17	3	tr
CAVIAR				
black granular	1 tbsp	40	1	3
black granular	1 oz	71	1	5
red granular	1 tbsp	40	1	3
red granular	1 oz	71	1	5
CELERIAC				
FRESH				
cooked	3½ oz	25	6	tr
raw	½ cup	31	7	tr

FOOD	PORTION	CALORIES	CHO	FAT

CELERY

DRIED
seed	1 tsp	8	1	tr

FRESH
diced, cooked	½ cup	11	3	tr
raw	1 stalk (2 oz)	6	1	tr
raw; diced	½ cup	9	2	tr

CELTUCE

raw	3½ oz	22	4	tr

CEREAL

COOKED
farina, dry	1 tbsp	40	9	0
farina; cooked	¾ cup	87	19	tr
oatmeal, instant; cooked w/o salt	1 cup	145	25	2
oatmeal, quick; cooked w/o salt	1 cup	145	25	2
oatmeal, regular; cooked w/o salt	1 cup	145	25	2
oatmeal, dry	1 cup	311	54	5
oatmeal; cooked	1 cup	145	25	2

READY-TO-EAT
all bran	⅓ cup (1 oz)	70	21	1
bran flakes	¾ cup (1 oz)	90	22	1
corn flakes	1¼ cup (1 oz)	110	24	tr
shredded wheat	⅔ cup (1 oz)	100	23	1

FOOD	PORTION	CALORIES	CHO	FAT
*sugar-coated corn flakes	¾ cup (1 oz)	110	26	1

CHAYOTE

FRESH
cooked	1 cup	38	8	1
raw	1 (7 oz)	49	11	1
raw; cut up	1 cup	32	7	tr

CHEESE

NATURAL
Bel Paese	3½ oz	391	0	30
blue	1 oz	100	1	8
blue; crumbled	1 cup	477	3	39
brick	1 oz	105	1	8
Brie	1 oz	95	tr	8
Camembert	1 oz	85	tr	7
Camembert	1 wedge (1⅓ oz)	114	tr	9
caraway	1 oz	107	1	8
cheddar	1 oz	114	tr	9
cheddar; shredded	1 cup	455	1	37
Cheshire	1 oz	110	1	9
colby	1 oz	112	1	9
Edam	1 oz	101	tr	8
Emmentaler	3½ oz	403	tr	30
feta	1 oz	75	1	6

FOOD	PORTION	CALORIES	CHO	FAT
fontina	1 oz	110	tr	9
gjetost	1 oz	132	12	8
Gorgonzola	3½ oz	376	1	31
Gouda	1 oz	101	1	8
Gruyère	1 oz	117	tr	9
Limburger	1 oz	93	tr	8
Monterey	1 oz	106	tr	9
mozzarella	1 oz	80	1	6
mozzarella	1 lb	1276	10	98
mozzarella, low moisture	1 oz	90	1	7
mozzarella, part skim	1 oz	72	1	5
mozzarella, part skim, low moisture	1 oz	79	1	5
Muenster	1 oz	104	tr	9
Parmesan, hard	1 oz	111	1	7
Parmesan; grated	1 tbsp	23	tr	2
Parmesan; grated	1 oz	129	1	9
Port du salut	1 oz	100	tr	8
provolone	1 oz	100	1	8
quark, 20% fat	3½ oz	116	3	5
quark, 40% fat	3½ oz	167	3	11
quark, made w/ skim milk	3½ oz	78	4	tr
ricotta	½ cup	216	4	16
ricotta	1 cup	428	7	32
ricotta, part skim	½ cup	171	6	10

FOOD	PORTION	CALORIES	CHO	FAT
ricotta, part skim	1 cup	340	13	19
Romadur, 40% fat	3½ oz	289	tr	20
Romano	1 oz	110	1	8
Roquefort	1 oz	105	1	9
Swiss	1 oz	107	1	8
Tilsit	1 oz	96	1	7
PROCESSED				
American	1 oz	106	tr	9
American, cheese food	1 oz	93	2	7
American, cheese food	1 pkg (8 oz)	745	17	56
American, cheese food, cold pack	1 oz	94	2	7
American, cheese food, cold pack	1 pkg (8 oz)	752	19	56
American, cheese spread	1 oz	82	2	6
American, cheese spread	1 jar (5 oz)	412	12	30
pimento	1 oz	106	tr	9
Swiss	1 oz	95	1	7
Swiss, cheese food	1 oz	92	1	7
Swiss, cheese food	1 pkg (8oz)	734	10	55

CHERIMOYA

fresh	1	515	131	2

CHERRIES

CANNED				
*sour in heavy syrup	½ cup	232	60	tr

FOOD	PORTION	CALORIES	CHO	FAT
*sour in light syrup	½ cup	189	49	tr
sour, water pack	1 cup	87	22	tr
*sweet in heavy syrup	½ cup	107	27	tr
*sweet in light syrup	½ cup	85	22	tr
sweet, juice pack	½ cup	68	17	tr
sweet, water pack	½ cup	57	15	tr
FRESH				
sour	1 cup	51	13	tr
sweet	10	49	11	1
FROZEN				
sour unsweetened	1 cup	72	17	1
*sweet sweetened	1 cup	232	58	tr

CHERVIL

seed	1 tsp	1	tr	tr

CHESTNUTS

Chinese dried	1 oz	103	23	tr
Chinese, raw	1 oz	64	14	tr
Chinese; cooked	1 oz	44	10	tr
Chinese; roasted	1 oz	68	15	tr
cooked	1 oz	37	8	tr
dried; peeled	1 oz	105	22	1
Japanese, dried	1 oz	102	23	tr
Japanese, raw	1 oz	44	10	tr
Japanese; roasted	1 oz	57	13	tr

FOOD	PORTION	CALORIES	CHO	FAT
Japanese; cooked	1 oz	16	4	tr
raw; peeled	1 oz	56	13	tr
roasted	1 oz	70	15	1
roasted	1 cup	350	76	3

CHIA SEEDS

dried	1 oz	134	14	7

CHICKEN

CANNED

chicken spread	1 tbsp	25	1	2
chicken spread	1 oz	55	2	3
chicken spread, barbecue flavored	1 oz	55	2	3
w/ broth	1 can (5 oz)	234	0	11
w/ broth	½ can (2.5 oz)	117	0	6

FRESH

broiler/fryer breast w/ skin; batter dipped, fried	½ breast (4.9 oz)	364	13	18
broiler/fryer thigh w/ skin; roasted	1 (2.2 oz)	153	0	10
broiler/fryer back meat w/o skin, raw	1 oz	42	0	2
broiler/fryer back w/ skin, raw	½ back (3.5 oz)	316	0	28
broiler/fryer back w/ skin; batter dipped, fried	½ back (2.5 oz)	238	7	16

FOOD	PORTION	CALORIES	CHO	FAT
broiler/fryer back w/ skin; floured, fried	1.5 oz	146	3	9
broiler/fryer back w/ skin; roasted	1 oz	96	0	7
broiler/fryer back w/ skin; stewed	½ back (2.1 oz)	158	0	11
broiler/fryer back w/o skin; fried	½ back (2 oz)	167	3	9
broiler/fryer breast w/ skin, raw	3.1 oz	150	0	8
broiler/fryer breast w/ skin; batter dipped, fried	2.9 oz	218	8	11
broiler/fryer breast w/ skin; roasted	½ breast (3.4 oz)	193	0	8
broiler/fryer breast w/ skin; roasted	2 oz	115	0	5
broiler/fryer breast w/ skin; stewed	½ breast (3.9 oz)	202	0	8
broiler/fryer breast w/o skin, raw	½ breast (4 oz)	129	0	1
broiler/fryer breast w/o skin; fried	½ breast (3 oz)	161	tr	4
broiler/fryer breast w/o skin; roasted	½ breast (3 oz)	142	0	3
broiler/fryer breast w/o skin; stewed	2 oz	86	0	2
broiler/fryer breast w/ skin, raw	½ breast (5.1 oz)	250	0	13
broiler/fryer dark meat w/ skin, raw	½ chicken (9.3 oz)	630	0	49

FOOD	PORTION	CALORIES	CHO	FAT
broiler/fryer dark meat w/ skin; batter dripped, fried	5.9 oz	497	16	31
broiler/fryer dark meat w/ skin; floured, fried	3.9 oz	313	4	19
broiler/fryer dark meat w/ skin; roasted	3.5 oz	256	0	16
broiler/fryer dark meat w/ skin; stewed	3.9 oz	256	0	16
broiler/fryer dark meat w/o skin, raw	3.8 oz	136	0	5
broiler/fryer dark meat w/o skin; fried	1 cup (5 oz)	334	4	16
broiler/fryer dark meat w/o skin; roasted	1 cup (5 oz)	286	0	14
broiler/fryer dark meat w/o skin; stewed	1 cup (5 oz)	269	0	13
broiler/fryer dark meat w/o skin; stewed	3 oz	165	0	8
broiler/fryer drumstick w/ skin, raw	1 (2.6 oz)	117	0	6
broiler/fryer drumstick w/ skin; batter dipped, fried	1 (2.6 oz)	193	6	11
broiler/fryer drumstick w/ skin; floured, fried	1 (1.7 oz)	120	1	7
broiler/fryer drumstick w/ skin; roasted	1 (1.8 oz)	112	0	6
broiler/fryer drumstick w/ skin; stewed	1 (2 oz)	116	0	6
broiler/fryer drumstick w/o skin, raw	1 (2.2 oz)	74	0	2

FOOD	PORTION	CALORIES	CHO	FAT
broiler/fryer drumstick w/o skin; fried	1 (1.5 oz)	82	0	3
broiler/fryer drumstick w/o skin; roasted	1 (1.5 oz)	76	0	2
broiler/fryer drumstick w/o skin; stewed	1 (1.6 oz)	78	0	3
broiler/fryer leg w/ skin, raw	1 (5.6 oz)	312	0	20
broiler/fryer leg w/ skin; batter dipped, fried	1 (5.5 oz)	431	14	26
broiler/fryer leg w/ skin; roasted	1 (4 oz)	265	0	15
broiler/fryer leg w/ skin; stewed	1 (4.4 oz)	275	0	16
broiler/fryer leg w/o skin, raw	1 (4.6 oz)	156	0	5
broiler/fryer leg w/o skin; fried	1 (3.3 oz)	195	1	9
broiler/fryer leg w/o skin; roasted	1 (3.3 oz)	182	0	8
broiler/fryer leg w/o skin; stewed	1 (3.5 oz)	187	0	8
broiler/fryer leg w/ skin; floured, fried	1 (3.9 oz)	285	3	16
broiler/fryer light meat w/ skin, raw	½ chicken (6.8 oz)	362	0	21
broiler/fryer light meat w/ skin, raw	4.1 oz	216	0	13
broiler/fryer light meat w/ skin; batter dipped, fried	4 oz	312	11	17

FOOD	PORTION	CALORIES	CHO	FAT
broiler/fryer light meat w/ skin; floured, fried	2.7 oz	192	1	9
broiler/fryer light meat w/ skin; roasted	2.8 oz	175	0	9
broiler/fryer light meat w/ skin; stewed	3.2 oz	181	0	9
broiler/fryer light meat w/o skin, raw	3.1 oz	100	0	1
broiler/fryer light meat w/o skin; fried	1 cup (5 oz)	268	1	8
broiler/fryer light meat w/o skin; roasted	1 cup (5 oz)	242	0	6
broiler/fryer light meat w/o skin; stewed	1 cup (5 oz)	223	0	6
broiler/fryer neck w/ skin, raw	1 (1.8 oz)	148	0	13
broiler/fryer neck w/ skin; stewed	1 (1.3 oz)	94	0	7
broiler/fryer neck w/o skin, raw	1 (.7 oz)	31	0	2
broiler/fryer neck w/o skin; stewed	1 (.6 oz)	32	0	1
broiler/fryer skin, raw	from ½ chicken (2.8 oz)	275	0	26
broiler/fryer skin; batter dipped, fried	from ½ chicken (6.7 oz)	748	44	55
broiler/fryer skin; batter dipped, fried	4 oz	449	26	33

FOOD	PORTION	CALORIES	CHO	FAT
broiler/fryer skin; floured, fried	1 oz	166	3	14
broiler/fryer skin; floured, fried	from ½ chicken (2 oz)	281	5	24
broiler/fryer skin; roasted	from ½ chicken (2 oz)	254	0	23
broiler/fryer skin; stewed	from ½ chicken (2.5 oz)	261	0	24
broiler/fryer thigh w/ skin; floured, fried	1 (2.2 oz)	162	2	9
broiler/fryer thigh w/ skin, raw	1 (3.3 oz)	199	0	14
broiler/fryer thigh w/ skin; batter dipped, fried	1 (3 oz)	238	8	14
broiler/fryer thigh w/ skin; stewed	1 (2.4 oz)	158	0	10
broiler/fryer thigh w/o skin, raw	1 (2.4 oz)	82	0	3
broiler/fryer thigh w/o skin; fried	1 (1.8 oz)	113	1	5
broiler/fryer thigh w/o skin; roasted	1 (1.8 oz)	109	0	6
broiler/fryer thigh w/o skin; stewed	1 (1.9 oz)	107	0	5
broiler/fryer w/ skin; floured, fried	½ breast (3.4 oz)	218	2	9

FOOD	PORTION	CALORIES	CHO	FAT
broiler/fryer w/o skin, raw	½ chicken (11.5 oz)	392	0	10
broiler/fryer w/o skin; roasted	1 cup (5 oz)	266	0	10
broiler/fryer w/o skin; fried	1 cup	307	2	13
broiler/fryer w/o skin; stewed	1 cup (5 oz)	248	0	9
broiler/fryer w/o skin; stewed	1 oz	54	0	3
broiler/fryer wing w/ skin, raw	1 (1.7 oz)	109	0	8
broiler/fryer wing w/ skin; batter dipped, fried	1 (1.7 oz)	159	5	11
broiler/fryer wing w/ skin; floured, fried	1 (1.1 oz)	103	1	7
broiler/fryer wing w/ skin; roasted	1 (1.2 oz)	99	0	7
broiler/fryer wing w/ skin; stewed	1 (1.4 oz)	100	0	7
broiler/fryer w/ skin, neck & giblets, raw	1 chicken (2.3 lbs)	2223	1	155
broiler/fryer w/ skin, neck & giblets; batter dipped, fried	1 chicken (2.3 lbs)	2987	93	180
broiler/fryer w/ skin, neck & giblets; roasted	1 chicken (1.5 lbs)	1598	tr	90
broiler/fryer w/ skin, neck & giblets; stewed	1 chicken (1.6 lbs)	1625	tr	93

FOOD	PORTION	CALORIES	CHO	FAT
broiler/fryer w/ skin, raw	½ chicken (16.1 oz)	990	0	69
broiler/fryer w/ skin; floured, fried	½ chicken (11 oz)	844	10	47
broiler/fryer w/ skin; fried	½ chicken (16.4 oz)	1347	44	81
broiler/fryer w/ skin; roasted	½ chicken (10.5 oz)	715	0	41
broiler/fryer w/ skin; stewed	½ chicken (11.7 oz)	730	0	42
capon w/ skin, neck & giblets, raw	1 chicken (4.7 lbs)	4987	2	364
capon w/ skin, neck & giblets; roasted	1 chicken (3.1 lbs)	3211	1	165
roaster dark meat w/o skin; roasted	1 cup (5 oz)	250	0	12
roaster light meat w/o skin; roasted	1 cup (5 oz)	214	0	6
roaster w/ skin, neck & giblets, raw	1 chicken (3.3 lbs)	3210	1	233
roaster w/ skin, neck & giblets; roasted	1 chicken (2.4 lbs)	2363	1	140
roaster w/o skin; roasted	1 cup (5 oz)	469	0	28
roaster w/ skin; roasted	½ chicken (1.1 lbs)	1071	0	64
stewing dark meat w/o skin; stewed	1 cup (5 oz)	361	0	21
stewing w/ skin, neck & giblets, raw	1 chicken (2 lbs)	2275	2	177

FOOD	PORTION	CALORIES	CHO	FAT
stewing w/ skin, neck & giblets; stewed	1 chicken (1.3 lbs)	1636	tr	107
stewing w/ skin; stewed	½ chicken (9.2 oz)	744	0	49
stewing w/ skin; stewed	6.2 oz	507	0	34
READY-TO-USE				
chicken roll, light meat	2 oz	90	1	4
chicken roll, light meat	1 pkg (6 oz)	271	4	13
poultry salad sandwich spread	1 tbsp	109	1	2
poultry salad sandwich spread	1 oz	238	2	4
TAKE OUT				
boneless, w/ barbecue sauce; breaded & fried	6 pieces (4.6 oz)	330	25	18
boneless, w/ honey; breaded & fried	6 pieces (4 oz)	339	27	18
boneless, w/ mustard sauce; breaded & fried	6 pieces (4.6 oz)	323	21	17
boneless, w/ sweet & sour sauce; breaded & fried	6 pieces (4.6 oz)	346	29	18
breast & wing; breaded & fried	2 pieces (5.7 oz)	494	20	30
drumstick; breaded & fried	2 pieces (5.2 oz)	430	16	27
fillet sandwich w/ cheese, mayonnaise, tomato, lettuce	1	632	42	39
fillet sandwich, plain	1	515	39	29
thigh; breaded & fried	2 pieces (5.2 oz)	430	16	27

FOOD	PORTION	CALORIES	CHO	FAT

CHICKEN DISHES

HOME RECIPE

FOOD	PORTION	CALORIES	CHO	FAT
chicken & noodles	1 cup	365	26	18
chicken à la king	1 cup	470	12	34

CHICKPEAS

CANNED

FOOD	PORTION	CALORIES	CHO	FAT
chickpeas	1 cup	285	54	3

DRIED

FOOD	PORTION	CALORIES	CHO	FAT
cooked	1 cup	269	45	4
raw	1 cup	729	121	12

CHICORY

FRESH

FOOD	PORTION	CALORIES	CHO	FAT
greens, raw; chopped	½ cup	21	4	tr
roots, raw; cut up	½ cup	33	8	tr
witloof, raw	½ cup	7	1	tr

CHILI

CANNED

FOOD	PORTION	CALORIES	CHO	FAT
chili w/ beans	1 cup	286	30	14

DRIED

FOOD	PORTION	CALORIES	CHO	FAT
powder	1 tsp	8	1	tr

TAKE-OUT

FOOD	PORTION	CALORIES	CHO	FAT
con carne w/ beans	8.9 oz	254	22	8

CHINESE PRESERVING MELON

FOOD	PORTION	CALORIES	CHO	FAT
cooked	½ cup	11	3	tr

FOOD	PORTION	CALORIES	CHO	FAT

CHIPS

POTATO

FOOD	PORTION	CALORIES	CHO	FAT
potato	10 chips	105	10	7
potato	1 oz	148	15	10
sticks	1 oz pkg	148	15	10
sticks	½ cup	94	10	6

CHITTERLINGS

pork; simmered	3 oz	258	0	24

CHIVES

DRIED

freeze-dried	1 tbsp	1	tr	tr

FRESH

raw; chopped	1 tbsp	1	tr	tr

CHOCOLATE

BAKING

*baking	1 oz	145	8	15

MIX

*powder	2–3 heaping tsp	75	20	1
*powder: as prep w/ whole milk	9 oz	226	31	9

SYRUP

*chocolate	1 cup	653	177	3
*chocolate	2 tbsp	82	22	tr
*chocolate; as prep w/ whole milk	9 oz	232	34	9

FOOD	PORTION	CALORIES	CHO	FAT
CINNAMON				
ground	1 tsp	6	2	tr
CISCO				
FRESH				
raw	3 oz	84	0	2
SMOKED				
smoked	3 oz	151	0	10
smoked	1 oz	50	0	3
CLAMS				
CANNED				
liquid only	1 cup	6	tr	tr
liquid only	3 oz	2	tr	tr
meat only	1 cup	236	8	3
meat only	3 oz	126	4	2
FRESH				
cooked	20 sm	133	5	2
cooked	3 oz	126	4	2
raw	3 oz	63	2	1
raw	9 lg	133	5	2
raw	20 sm	133	5	2
HOME RECIPE				
breaded & fried	3 oz	171	9	9
breaded & fried	20 sm	379	19	21
TAKE-OUT				
breaded & fried	¾ cup	451	39	26

FOOD	PORTION	CALORIES	CHO	FAT
CLOVES				
ground	1 tsp	7	1	tr
COCOA				
MIX				
*powder	1 oz	102	23	1
PREPARED				
*home recipe	1 cup	218	26	9
*hot cocoa	1 cup	218	26	9
mix w/ Nutrasweet; as prep w/ water	7 oz	48	9	tr
*mix; as prep w/ water	7 oz	103	23	1
COCONUT				
coconut water	1 tbsp	3	1	tr
coconut water	1 cup	46	9	tr
*cream, canned	1 tbsp	36	2	3
*cream, canned	1 cup	568	25	52
*dried, sweetened, flaked	7 oz pkg	944	95	64
*dried, sweetened, flaked	1 cup	351	35	24
*dried, sweetened, flaked, canned	1 cup	341	32	24
*dried, sweetened, shredded	7 oz pkg	997	95	71
*dried, sweetened, shredded	1 cup	466	44	33
dried, toasted	1 oz	168	13	13
dried, unsweetened	1 oz	187	7	18
milk, canned	1 tbsp	30	tr	3

FOOD	PORTION	CALORIES	CHO	FAT
milk, canned	1 cup	445	6	48
milk, frozen	1 tbsp	30	1	3
milk, frozen	1 cup	486	13	50
raw; shredded	1 cup	283	12	27

COD

CANNED				
Atlantic	3 oz	89	0	1
Atlantic	1 can (11 oz)	327	0	3
DRIED				
Atlantic	3 oz	246	0	2
FRESH				
Atlantic, raw	3 oz	70	0	1
Atlantic; cooked	1 fillet (6.3 oz)	189	0	2
Atlantic; cooked	3 oz	89	0	1
Pacific, raw	3 oz	70	0	1

COFFEE

INSTANT				
*cappuccino mix; as prep w/ water	7 oz	62	11	2
decaffeinated	1 rounded tsp	4	1	0
decaffeinated; as prep w/ water	6 oz	4	1	0
*French mix; as prep w/ water	7 oz	57	7	3

FOOD	PORTION	CALORIES	CHO	FAT
*mocha mix; as prep w/ water	7 oz	51	8	2
regular	1 rounded tsp	4	1	0
regular w/ chicory	1 rounded tsp	6	1	0
regular w/ chicory; as prep w/ water	6 oz	6	1	0
regular; as prep w/ water	6 oz	4	1	0
REGULAR brewed	6 oz	4	1	0

COFFEE SUBSTITUTES

FOOD	PORTION	CALORIES	CHO	FAT
powder	1 tsp	9	2	tr
powder; as prep w/ milk	6 oz	121	10	6
powder; as prep w/ water	6 oz	9	2	tr

COFFEE WHITENERS

FOOD	PORTION	CALORIES	CHO	FAT
LIQUID nondairy, frzn	1 tbsp	20	2	2
POWDER nondairy	1 tsp	11	1	tr

COLLARDS

FOOD	PORTION	CALORIES	CHO	FAT
FRESH cooked	½ cup	13	3	tr
raw; chopped	½ cup	18	4	tr
FROZEN chopped; cooked	½ cup	31	6	tr

FOOD	PORTION	CALORIES	CHO	FAT

COOKIES

HOME RECIPE

FOOD	PORTION	CALORIES	CHO	FAT
*chocolate chip	4 (1½ oz)	185	26	11
*peanut butter	4 (1.7 oz)	245	28	14
*shortbread	2 (1 oz)	145	17	8
READY-TO-EAT				
*animal crackers	1 box (2.4 oz)	299	51	9
*chocolate chip	4 (1½ oz)	180	28	9
*chocolate chip	1 box (1.9 oz)	233	36	12
*chocolate sandwich	4 (1.4 oz)	195	29	8
*fig bars	4 (2 oz)	210	42	4
*graham	2 squares	60	11	1
*oatmeal raisin	4 (1.8 oz)	245	36	10
*shortbread	4 (1 oz)	155	20	8
*vanilla sandwich	4 (1.4 oz)	195	29	8
*vanilla wafers	10 (1.3 oz)	185	29	7
REFRIGERATED				
*chocolate chip	4 (1.7 oz)	225	32	11
*sugar	4 (1.7 oz)	235	31	12

CORIANDER

FOOD	PORTION	CALORIES	CHO	FAT
leaf, dried	1 tsp	2	tr	tr
seed	1 tsp	5	1	tr
FRESH				
coriander	¼ cup	1	tr	tr

FOOD	PORTION	CALORIES	CHO	FAT

CORN

CANNED

FOOD	PORTION	CALORIES	CHO	FAT
cream style	½ cup	93	23	1
w/ red & green peppers	½ cup	86	21	1
white	½ cup	66	15	1
yellow	½ cup	66	15	1

FRESH

FOOD	PORTION	CALORIES	CHO	FAT
on-the-cob w/ butter; cooked	1 ear	155	32	3
white, raw	½ cup	66	15	1
white; cooked	½ cup	89	21	1
yellow, raw	½ cup	66	15	1
yellow, raw	1 ear (3 oz)	77	17	1
yellow, cooked	1 ear (2.7 oz)	83	19	1
yellow; cooked	½ cup	89	21	1

FROZEN

FOOD	PORTION	CALORIES	CHO	FAT
cooked	½ cup	67	17	tr
on-the-cob; cooked	1 ear (2.2 oz)	59	14	tr

CORNMEAL

FOOD	PORTION	CALORIES	CHO	FAT
corn grits, uncooked	1 cup	579	124	2
corn grits; cooked	1 cup	146	31	tr
degermed	1 cup	506	107	2
self-rising, degermed	1 cup	489	103	2
whole grain	1 cup	442	94	4

FOOD	PORTION	CALORIES	CHO	FAT
CORNSTARCH				
cornstarch	⅓ cup	164	39	tr
cornstarch	3½ oz	346	86	8
COTTAGE CHEESE				
REDUCED CALORIE				
lowfat, 1%	4 oz	82	3	1
lowfat, 1%	1 cup	164	6	2
lowfat, 2%	4 oz	101	4	2
lowfat, 2%	1 cup	203	8	4
REGULAR				
creamed	4 oz	117	3	5
creamed	1 cup	217	6	9
dry curd	1 cup	123	3	1
dry curd	4 oz	96	2	tr
COTTONSEED				
kernels, roasted	1 tbsp	51	2	4
COUSCOUS				
cooked	½ cup	101	21	tr
dry	½ cup	346	71	tr
COWPEAS				
CANNED				
common	1 cup	184	33	1
common w/ pork	½ cup	199	40	4

FOOD	PORTION	CALORIES	CHO	FAT
DRIED				
catjang, raw	1 cup	572	100	3
catjang; cooked	1 cup	200	35	1
common, raw	1 cup	562	100	2
common; cooked	1 cup	198	36	1
FRESH				
leafy tips, raw; chopped	1 cup	10	2	tr
leafy tips; chopped, cooked	1 cup	12	1	tr
FROZEN				
cooked	½ cup	112	20	tr

CRAB

FOOD	PORTION	CALORIES	CHO	FAT
CANNED				
blue	3 oz	84	0	1
blue	1 cup	133	0	2
FRESH				
Alaska king, raw	1 leg (6 oz)	144	0	1
Alaska king, raw	3 oz	71	0	1
Alaska king; cooked	1 leg (4.7 oz)	129	0	2
Alaska king; cooked	3 oz	82	0	1
blue, raw	3 oz	74	tr	1
blue, raw	1 crab (.7 oz)	18	tr	tr
blue: cooked	3 oz	87	0	2
blue; cooked	1 cup	138	0	2
Dungeness, raw	1 crab (5.7 oz)	140	1	2
Dungeness, raw	3 oz	73	1	1

FOOD	PORTION	CALORIES	CHO	FAT
queen, raw	3 oz	76	0	1
READY-TO-USE				
crab cakes	1 cake (2.1 oz)	93	tr	5
TAKE-OUT				
baked	1 (2 oz)	88	2	1
cake	1 (3.8 oz)	290	9	19
soft-shell; fried	1 (4.4 oz)	334	31	18

CRACKERS

FOOD	PORTION	CALORIES	CHO	FAT
cheese	10 (⅓ oz)	50	6	3
crispbread	3½ oz	317	65	1
melba toast, plain	1	20	4	tr
peanut butter sandwich	1 (⅓ oz)	40	5	2
saltines	4	50	9	1
zwieback	3½ oz	374	73	4

CRANBERRIES

FOOD	PORTION	CALORIES	CHO	FAT
CANNED				
*cranberry sauce, sweetened	½ cup	209	54	tr
FRESH				
chopped	1 cup	54	14	tr
JUICE				
*cranberry juice cocktail	1 cup	147	38	tr
*cranberry juice cocktail	6 oz	108	27	tr
*cranberry juice cocktail, frzn	12 oz	821	210	0
*cranberry juice cocktail, frzn; as prep	6 oz	102	26	0

FOOD	PORTION	CALORIES	CHO	FAT
low calorie cranberry juice cocktail	6 oz	33	9	0

CRANBERRY BEANS

CANNED				
cranberry beans	1 cup	216	39	1
DRIED				
cooked	1 cup	240	43	1
raw	1 cup	652	117	2

CRAYFISH

FRESH				
cooked	3 oz	97	0	1
raw	3 oz	76	0	1
raw	8	24	0	tr

CREAM

LIQUID				
half & half	1 tbsp	20	1	2
half & half	1 cup	315	10	28
heavy whipping	1 tbsp	52	tr	6
light whipping	1 tbsp	44	tr	5
light, coffee	1 tbsp	29	1	3
light, coffee	1 cup	496	9	46
WHIPPED				
heavy whipping	1 cup	411	7	44
light whipping	1 cup	345	7	37

FOOD	PORTION	CALORIES	CHO	FAT

CREAM CHEESE

NEUFCHATEL

Neufchatel	1 oz	74	1	7
Neufchatel	1 pkg (3 oz)	221	3	20

REGULAR

cream cheese	1 oz	99	1	10
cream cheese	1 pkg (3 oz)	297	2	30

CRESS

FRESH

garden, raw	½ cup	8	1	tr
garden; cooked	½ cup	16	3	tr

CROAKER

Atlantic, raw	3 oz	89	0	3
Atlantic; breaded & fried	3 oz	188	6	11

CROISSANT

croissant	1 (2 oz)	235	27	12

TAKE-OUT

w/ egg & cheese	1	369	24	25
w/ egg, cheese & bacon	1	413	24	28
w/ egg, cheese & ham	1	475	24	34
w/ egg, cheese & sausage	1	524	25	38

CUCUMBER

FRESH

raw	1 (11 oz)	39	9	tr

FOOD	PORTION	CALORIES	CHO	FAT
raw; sliced	½ cup	7	2	tr

CUMIN
seed	1 tsp	8	1	tr

CURRANTS

DRIED
zante	½ cup	204	53	tr

FRESH
black	½ cup	36	9	tr

JUICE
black currant nectar	3½ oz	55	13	0
red currant nectar	3½ oz	54	13	tr

CUSK

FRESH
raw	3 oz	74	0	1

CUSTARD
*baked	1 cup	305	29	17

CUTTLEFISH

FRESH
raw	3 oz	67	1	1

DANDELION GREENS
cooked	½ cup	17	3	tr
raw; chopped	½ cup	13	3	tr

FOOD	PORTION	CALORIES	CHO	FAT
DANISH PASTRY				
*cheese	1 (3 oz)	353	29	25
*cinnamon	1 (3 oz)	349	47	17
*fruit	1 (2.3 oz)	235	28	13
*fruit	1 (3.3 oz)	335	45	16
*plain	1 (2 oz)	220	26	12
*plain ring	1 (12 oz)	1305	152	71
DATES				
DRIED				
chopped	1 cup	489	131	1
whole	10	228	61	tr
DILL				
seed	1 tsp	6	1	tr
weed, dried	1 tsp	3	1	tr
DOCK				
FRESH				
cooked	3½ oz	20	3	1
raw; chopped	½ cup	15	2	tr
DOGFISH				
raw	3½ oz	193	0	15
DOLPHINFISH				
FRESH				
raw	3 oz	73	0	1

FOOD	PORTION	CALORIES	CHO	FAT
DOUGHNUTS				
cake type	1 (1.8 oz)	210	24	12
glazed	1 (2 oz)	235	26	13
DRINK MIXER				
whiskey sour mix	2 oz	55	14	0
DRUM				
FRESH				
freshwater, raw	3 oz	101	0	4
DUCK				
w/ skin, raw	½ duck (1.4 lbs)	2561	0	249
w/ skin; roasted	6 oz	583	0	49
w/ skin; roasted	½ duck (13.4 oz)	1287	0	108
w/o skin, raw	4.8 oz	180	0	8
w/o skin; roasted	3.5 oz	201	0	11
w/o skin; roasted	½ duck (7.8 oz)	445	0	25
wild breast w/o skin, raw	½ breast (2.9 oz)	102	0	4
wild w/ skin, raw	½ duck (9.5 oz)	571	0	41
DURIAN				
fresh	3½ oz	141	29	2

FOOD	PORTION	CALORIES	CHO	FAT
EEL				
FRESH				
cooked	3 oz	200	0	13
cooked	1 fillet (5.6 oz)	375	0	24
raw	3 oz	156	0	10
EGG				
CHICKEN				
fried w/ margarine	1	91	1	7
frozen	1	75	1	5
frozen	1 cup	363	3	24
hard cooked	1	77	1	5
hard cooked; chopped	1 cup	210	2	14
poached	1	74	1	5
raw	1	75	1	5
raw	1 cup	363	3	24
scrambled w/ whole milk & margarine	1	101	1	7
scrambled w/ whole milk & margarine	1 cup	365	5	27
scrambled, plain	2	200	2	15
white only	1	17	tr	0
white only	1 cup	121	2	0
yolk, raw	1 cup	870	4	75
yolk, raw	1	59	tr	5

FOOD	PORTION	CALORIES	CHO	FAT
OTHER POULTRY				
duck, raw	1	130	1	10
goose, raw	1	267	2	19
quail, raw	1	14	tr	1
turkey, raw	1	135	1	9

EGG DISHES

TAKE-OUT				
sandwich w/ cheese, ham	1	348	31	16
sandwich w/ cheese	1	340	26	19

EGG SUBSTITUTES

frozen	¼ cup	96	2	7
frozen	1 cup	384	8	27
liquid	1½ oz	40	tr	2
liquid	1 cup	211	2	8
powder	0.7 oz	88	4	3
powder	0.35 oz	44	2	1

EGGNOG

*eggnog	1 cup	342	34	19
*eggnog	1 qt	1368	138	76
*eggnog flavor mix; as prep w/ milk	9 oz	260	39	8

FOOD	PORTION	CALORIES	CHO	FAT

EGGPLANT

FRESH

| cubed, cooked | ½ cup | 13 | 3 | tr |
| raw, cut up | ½ cup | 11 | 3 | tr |

ELDERBERRIES

| elderberries | 1 cup | 105 | 27 | 1 |

JUICE

| elderberry | 3½ oz | 38 | 8 | 0 |

ELK

| raw | 1 oz | 32 | 0 | tr |
| roasted | 3 oz | 124 | 0 | 2 |

ENDIVE

| fresh | 3½ oz | 9 | tr | tr |

FRESH

| raw; chopped | ½ cup | 4 | 1 | tr |

ENGLISH MUFFIN

| plain; toasted | 1 | 140 | 27 | 1 |

TAKE-OUT

w/ butter	1	189	30	6
w/ cheese & sausage	1	394	29	24
w/ egg, cheese & bacon	1	487	31	31
w/ egg, cheese & canadian bacon	1	383	31	20

FOOD	PORTION	CALORIES	CHO	FAT
EPPAW				
raw	½ cup	75	16	1
FALAFEL				
falafel	1 (1.2 oz)	57	5	3
falafel	3 (1.8 oz)	170	16	9
FAT				
beef suet, raw	1 oz	242	0	27
beef tallow	1 tbsp	115	0	13
beef, raw	1 oz	191	0	20
beef; cooked	1 oz	193	0	20
chicken	1 cup	1846	0	205
chicken	1 tbsp	115	0	13
chicken, raw	1 oz	201	0	22
cocoa butter	1 tbsp	120	0	14
duck	1 tbsp	115	0	13
goose	1 tbsp	115	0	13
lamb, New Zealand, raw	1 oz	182	0	19
lard	1 cup	1849	0	205
lard	1 tbsp	115	0	13
nutmeg butter	1 tbsp	120	0	14
pork; cooked	1 oz	200	0	21
salt pork	1 oz	212	0	23
shortening	1 tbsp	113	0	13

FOOD	PORTION	CALORIES	CHO	FAT
turkey	1 tbsp	115	0	13
ucuhuba butter	1 tbsp	120	0	14

FENNEL

seed	1 tsp	7	1	tr

FENUGREEK

seed	1 tsp	12	2	tr

FIGS

CANNED				
*in heavy syrup	3	75	19	tr
*in light syrup	3	58	15	tr
water pack	3	42	11	tr
DRIED				
cooked	½ cup	140	16	1
whole	10	477	122	2
FRESH				
fig	1 med	50	10	tr

FILBERTS

dried, unblanched	1 oz	179	4	18
dried, blanched	1 oz	191	5	19
dry roasted, unblanched	1 oz	188	5	19
oil roasted, unblanched	1 oz	187	5	18

FOOD	PORTION	CALORIES	CHO	FAT

FISH

FROZEN

| breaded fillet; as prep | 1 (2 oz) | 155 | 14 | 7 |
| sticks; as prep | 1 stick (1 oz) | 76 | 7 | 3 |

TAKE-OUT

| sandwich w/ tartar sauce | 1 | 431 | 41 | 55 |
| sandwich w/ tartar sauce, cheese | 1 | 524 | 48 | 29 |

FLATFISH

FRESH

cooked	1 fillet (4.5 oz)	148	0	2
cooked	3 oz	99	0	1
raw	3 oz	78	0	1

TAKE-OUT

| battered & fried | 3.2 oz | 211 | 15 | 11 |
| breaded & fried | 3.2 oz | 211 | 15 | 11 |

FLOUR

corn, masa	1 cup	416	87	4
corn, whole grain	1 cup	422	90	5
cottonseed, lowfat	1 oz	94	10	tr
peanut, defatted	1 cup	196	21	tr
peanut, defatted	1 oz	92	10	tr
peanut, lowfat	1 oz	120	9	6
peanut, lowfat	1 cup	257	19	13

FOOD	PORTION	CALORIES	CHO	FAT
potato	1 cup	628	143	1
rice, brown	1 cup	574	121	4
rice, white	1 cup	578	127	2
rye, dark	1 cup	415	88	3
rye, light	1 cup	374	82	1
rye, medium	1 cup	361	79	2
sesame, lowfat	1 oz	95	10	tr
triticale, whole grain	1 cup	440	95	2
white, all-purpose	1 cup	455	95	1
white, bread	1 cup	495	99	2
white, cake	1 cup	395	85	tr
white, self-rising	1 cup	442	93	1
whole wheat	1 cup	407	87	2

FRENCH BEANS

DRIED

cooked	1 cup	228	43	1
raw	1 cup	631	118	4

FRENCH TOAST

HOME RECIPE

French toast	1 slice	155	17	7

TAKE-OUT

w/ butter	2 slices	356	36	19

FOOD	PORTION	CALORIES	CHO	FAT

FRUIT DRINKS

FROZEN

FOOD	PORTION	CALORIES	CHO	FAT
*citrus juice drink	12 oz	684	171	tr
*citrus juice drink; as prep	1 cup	114	28	0
*fruit punch	1 can (12 oz)	678	173	tr
*fruit punch; as prep w/ water	1 cup	113	29	tr
*lemonade	1 can (6 oz)	397	103	tr
*lemonade; as prep w/ water	1 cup	100	26	tr
*limeade	1 can (6 oz)	408	108	tr
*limeade; as prep w/ water	1 cup	102	27	tr
MIX				
*fruit punch; as prep w/water	9 oz	97	25	0
lemonade powder w/ Nutrasweet; as prep w/ water	1 pitcher (67 oz)	40	10	0
*lemonade powder; as prep w/ water	9 oz	113	29	tr
READY-TO-USE				
*cranberry apricot drink	6 oz	118	30	0
*cranberry apple drink	6 oz	123	32	0
*fruit punch	6 oz	87	22	tr
*orange & apricot drink	1 cup	128	32	tr
orange & grapefruit juice	1 cup	107	25	tr
*pineapple & grapefruit drink	1 cup	117	29	tr
*pineapple & orange drink	1 cup	125	29	0

FOOD	PORTION	CALORIES	CHO	FAT

FRUIT, MIXED

CANNED

FOOD	PORTION	CALORIES	CHO	FAT
*fruit cocktail in heavy syrup	½ cup	93	24	tr
fruit cocktail, water pack	½ cup	40	10	tr
fruit cocktail, juice pack	½ cup	56	15	tr
fruit salad, juice pack	½ cup	62	16	tr
fruit salad, water pack	½ cup	37	10	tr
*fruit salad in heavy syrup	½ cup	94	24	tr
*fruit salad in light syrup	½ cup	73	19	tr
*mixed fruit in heavy syrup	½ cup	92	24	tr
*tropical fruit salad in heavy syrup	½ cup	110	29	tr

DRIED

FOOD	PORTION	CALORIES	CHO	FAT
mixed	11 oz pkg	712	188	1

FROZEN

FOOD	PORTION	CALORIES	CHO	FAT
*mixed fruit sweetened	1 cup	245	61	tr

GARLIC

FOOD	PORTION	CALORIES	CHO	FAT
powder	1 tsp	9	2	tr

FRESH

FOOD	PORTION	CALORIES	CHO	FAT
clove	1	4	1	tr

GEFILTE FISH

READY-TO-USE

FOOD	PORTION	CALORIES	CHO	FAT
sweet recipe	1 piece (1.5 oz)	35	3	1

FOOD	PORTION	CALORIES	CHO	FAT
GELATIN				
MIX				
*fruit flavored; as prep	½ cup	70	17	0
low calorie	½ cup	8	0	0
GIBLETS				
capon, raw	4 oz	150	2	6
capon; simmered	1 cup (5 oz)	238	0	8
chicken; floured, fried	1 cup (5 oz)	402	6	19
chicken; simmered	1 cup (5 oz)	228	1	7
chicken; raw	2.6 oz	93	1	3
turkey, raw	8.6 oz	314	5	10
turkey; simmered	1 cup (5 oz)	243	3	7
GINGER				
ground	1 tsp	6	1	tr
root, fresh	5 slices	8	2	tr
root, fresh	¼ cup	17	4	tr
GINKGO NUTS				
canned	1 oz	32	6	tr
dried	1 oz	99	21	tr
raw	1 oz	52	11	tr
GIZZARDS				
chicken; simmered	1 cup (5 oz)	222	2	5
chicken; raw	1 (1.3 oz)	41	tr	2

FOOD	PORTION	CALORIES	CHO	FAT
turkey, raw	1 (4 oz)	133	1	4
turkey; simmered	1 cup (5 oz)	236	1	6

GOAT

raw	1 oz	31	0	1
roasted	3 oz	122	0	3

GOOSE

FRESH

w/ skin, raw	½ goose (2.9 lb)	4893	0	443
w/ skin; roasted	6.6 oz	574	0	41
w/ skin; roasted	½ goose (1.7 lbs)	2362	0	170
w/o skin; roasted	5 oz	340	0	18
w/o skin; roasted	½ goose (1.3 lbs)	1406	0	75

GOOSEBERRIES

fresh	1 cup	67	15	1
CANNED				
*in light syrup	½ cup	93	24	tr

GRAPEFRUIT

juice pack	½ cup	46	11	tr
unsweetened	1 cup	93	22	tr
water pack	½ cup	44	11	tr
FRESH				
pink	½	37	9	tr

FOOD	PORTION	CALORIES	CHO	FAT
pink sections	1 cup	69	18	tr
red	½	37	9	tr
red sections	1 cup	69	18	tr
white	½	39	10	tr
white sections	1 cup	76	19	tr
JUICE				
fresh	1 cup	96	23	tr
frzn; as prep	1 cup	102	24	tr
frzn; not prep	6 oz	302	72	1
*sweetened	1 cup	116	28	tr

GRAPES

CANNED				
*Thompson seedless in heavy syrup	½ cup	94	25	tr
Thompson seedless, water pack	½ cup	48	13	tr
FRESH				
grapes	10	36	9	tr
JUICE				
bottled	1 cup	155	38	tr
*frzn sweetened; not prep	6 oz	386	96	1
*frzn, sweetened; as prep	1 cup	128	32	tr
*grape drink	6 oz	84	22	0

GRAVY

CANNED				
au jus	1 cup	38	6	tr

FOOD	PORTION	CALORIES	CHO	FAT
beef	1 cup	124	11	5
chicken	1 cup	189	13	14
mushroom	1 cup	120	13	6
turkey	1 cup	122	12	5
DRY				
au jus; as prep	1 cup	19	2	1
brown; as prep	1 cup	9	2	tr
chicken; as prep	1 cup	83	14	2
mushroom; as prep	1 cup	70	14	1
pork; as prep	1 cup	76	13	2
turkey; as prep	1 cup	87	15	2

GREAT NORTHERN BEANS

FOOD	PORTION	CALORIES	CHO	FAT
CANNED				
great northern	1 cup	300	55	1
DRIED				
cooked	1 cup	210	37	1
raw	1 cup	621	114	2

GROUNDCHERRIES

FOOD	PORTION	CALORIES	CHO	FAT
fresh	½ cup	37	8	tr

GROUPER

FOOD	PORTION	CALORIES	CHO	FAT
FRESH				
cooked	1 fillet (7.1 oz)	238	0	3
cooked	3 oz	100	0	1
raw	3 oz	78	0	1

FOOD	PORTION	CALORIES	CHO	FAT
GUAVA				
guava sauce	½ cup	43	11	tr
FRESH				
guava	1	45	11	1
GUINEA HEN				
w/ skin, raw	½ hen (12.1 oz)	545	0	22
w/o skin, raw	½ hen (9.3 oz)	292	0	7
HADDOCK				
cooked	1 fillet (5.3 oz)	168	0	1
cooked	3 oz	95	0	1
raw	3 oz	74	0	1
SMOKED				
smoked	3 oz	99	0	1
smoked	1 oz	33	0	tr
HAKE				
raw	3½ oz	84	0	1
HALIBUT				
FRESH				
Atlantic & Pacific, raw	3 oz	93	0	2
Atlantic & Pacific; cooked	3 oz	119	0	2
Atlantic & Pacific; cooked	½ fillet (5.6 oz)	223	0	5
Greenland, raw	3 oz	158	0	12

FOOD	PORTION	CALORIES	CHO	FAT

HAM

FOOD	PORTION	CALORIES	CHO	FAT
canned (13% fat); roasted	3 oz	192	tr	13
canned, extra lean (4% fat)	3 oz	116	tr	4
chopped	1 oz	65	0	5
chopped, canned	1 oz	68	tr	5
ham & cheese loaf	1 oz	73	1	6
ham & cheese spread	1 tbsp	37	tr	3
ham & cheese spread	1 oz	69	1	5
ham salad spread	1 tbsp	32	2	2
ham salad spread	1 oz	61	3	4
minced	1 oz	75	1	6
sliced, extra lean (5% fat)	1 oz	37	tr	1
sliced, regular (11% fat)	1 oz	52	1	3
steak, boneless, extra lean	1 oz	35	0	1

HAM DISHES

TAKE-OUT

FOOD	PORTION	CALORIES	CHO	FAT
sandwich w/ cheese	1	353	33	15

HAMBURGER

TAKE-OUT

FOOD	PORTION	CALORIES	CHO	FAT
double patty w/ bun, cheese	1 reg	457	22	28
double patty w/ bun	1 reg	544	43	28
double patty w/ bun, catsup, mayonnaise, mustard, pickle, onion, tomato	1 lg	540	40	27

FOOD	PORTION	CALORIES	CHO	FAT
double patty w/ bun, catsup, mustard, pickle, onion	1 reg	576	39	32
double patty w/ bun, cheese, catsup, mustard, mayonnaise, pickle, tomato	1 lg	706	40	44
double patty w/ bun, cheese, catsup, pickle, mayonnaise, onion, tomato	1 reg	416	35	21
double patty w/ double bun, catsup, pickle, mayonnaise, onion, tomato	1 reg	649	53	35
double patty w/ double bun, cheese	1 reg	461	44	22
single patty w/ bun	1 reg	275	31	12
single patty w/ bun	1 lg	400	25	23
single patty w/ bun, catsup, mayonnaise, mustard, pickle, onion, tomato	1 reg	279	27	13
single patty w/ bun, cheese	1 reg	320	32	15
single patty w/ bun, cheese	1 lg	608	47	33
single patty w/ bun, cheese, bacon, catsup, mustard, pickle, onion	1 lg	609	37	37
single patty w/ bun, cheese, ham, catsup, mayonnaise, pickle, tomato	1 lg	745	38	48
triple patty w/ bun, catsup, mustard, pickle	1 lg	693	29	41
triple patty w/ bun, cheese	1 lg	769	27	51

FOOD	PORTION	CALORIES	CHO	FAT
HEART				
beef; simmered	3 oz	148	tr	5
chicken; simmered	1 cup (5 oz)	268	tr	11
chicken; raw	1 (⅕ oz)	9	tr	1
lamb; braised	3 oz	158	2	7
turkey, raw	1 (1 oz)	41	tr	2
turkey; simmered	1 cup (5 oz)	257	3	9
veal; braised	3 oz	158	tr	6
HERBS/SPICES				
DRIED				
curry powder	1 tsp	6	1	tr
poultry seasoning	1 tsp	5	1	tr
pumpkin pie spice	1 tsp	6	1	tr
HERRING				
FRESH				
Atlantic, raw	3 oz	134	0	8
Atlantic; cooked	1 fillet (5 oz)	290	0	17
Atlantic; cooked	3 oz	172	0	10
Pacific, raw	3 oz	166	0	12
READY-TO-USE				
Atlantic kippered	1 fillet (1.4 oz)	87	0	5
Atlantic, pickled	½ oz	39	1	3
HICKORY NUTS				
dried	1 oz	187	5	18

FOOD	PORTION	CALORIES	CHO	FAT
HOMINY				
CANNED				
hominy	½ cup	57	11	tr
HONEY				
*honey	1 cup	1030	279	0
*honey	1 tbsp	65	17	0
HONEYDEW				
cubed	1 cup	60	16	tr
fresh	⅒	46	12	tr
HORSE				
raw	1 oz	38	0	1
roasted	3 oz	149	0	5
HOT DOG				
CHICKEN				
chicken	1 (1.5 oz)	116	3	9
MEAT				
beef	1 (2 oz)	184	1	17
beef	1 (1.6 oz)	145	1	13
beef & pork	1 (2 oz)	183	1	17
beef & pork	1 (1.6 oz)	144	1	13
TAKE-OUT				
corndog	1	460	56	19
w/ bun, chili	1	297	31	13
w/ bun, plain	1	242	18	15

FOOD	PORTION	CALORIES	CHO	FAT
TURKEY				
turkey	1 (1.5 oz)	102	1	8

HUMMUS

hummus	⅓ cup	140	17	7
hummus	1 cup	420	50	21

HYACINTH BEANS

DRIED				
cooked	1 cup	228	40	1
raw	1 cup	723	128	4

ICE CREAM AND FROZEN DESSERTS

*French vanilla, soft serve	1 cup	377	38	23
*French vanilla, soft serve	½ gal	3014	306	180
*orange sherbet	1 cup	270	59	4
*orange sherbet	½ gal	2158	469	31
*vanilla ice milk, soft serve	1 cup	223	38	5
*vanilla ice milk, soft serve	½ gal	1787	307	37
*vanilla ice milk	1 cup	184	29	6
*vanilla ice milk	½ gal	1469	232	45
*vanilla, 10% fat	1 cup	269	32	14
*vanilla, 10% fat	½ gal	2153	254	115
*vanilla, 16% fat	1 cup	349	32	24
*vanilla, 16% fat	½ gal	2805	256	190
TAKE-OUT				
*cone, vanilla, ice milk, soft serve	1 (4.6 oz)	164	24	6

FOOD	PORTION	CALORIES	CHO	FAT
*sundae, caramel	1 (5.4 oz)	303	49	9
*sundae, hot fudge	1 (5.4 oz)	284	48	9
*sundae, strawberry	1 (5.4 oz)	269	45	8

JACKFRUIT

fresh	3½ oz	70	4	tr

JAM/JELLY/PRESERVES

*apple jelly	3½ oz	259	65	0
*apricot jam	3½ oz	250	62	0
*blackberry jam	3½ oz	237	59	0
*cherry jam	3½ oz	250	62	0
diet jelly (artifically sweetened)	1 tbsp	6	1	tr
*orange jam	3½ oz	243	60	0
*plum jam	3½ oz	241	60	0
*quince jam	3½ oz	236	59	0
*raspberry jam	3½ oz	248	61	0
*raspberry jelly	3½ oz	259	65	0
*red current jelly	3½ oz	265	66	0
*red current jam	3½ oz	237	59	0
*rose hip jam	3½ oz	250	62	0
*strawberry jam	3½ oz	234	58	0

JAVA PLUM

fresh	1 cup	82	21	tr

FOOD	PORTION	CALORIES	CHO	FAT
JEW'S EAR				
pepeao, dried	½ cup	36	10	tr
pepeao, raw; sliced	1 cup	25	7	tr
JUJUBE				
fresh	3½ oz	105	24	tr
KALE				
FRESH				
chopped, cooked	½ cup	21	4	tr
raw; chopped	½ cup	21	3	tr
Scotch; chopped, cooked	½ cup	18	4	tr
FROZEN				
chopped, cooked	½ cup	20	4	tr
KEFIR				
kefir	3½ oz	66	5	4
KIDNEY				
beef; simmered	3 oz	122	0	3
lamb; braised	3 oz	117	1	3
veal; braised	3 oz	139	0	5
KIDNEY BEANS				
CANNED				
kidney beans	1 cup	208	38	1
red	1 cup	216	40	1
DRIED				
California red, raw	1 cup	609	110	tr

FOOD	PORTION	CALORIES	CHO	FAT
California red; cooked	1 cup	219	40	tr
kidney beans, raw	1 cup	613	110	2
kidney beans; cooked	1 cup	225	40	1
red, raw	1 cup	619	113	2
red; cooked	1 cup	225	40	1
royal red, raw	1 cup	605	107	1
royal red; cooked	1 cup	218	39	tr
SPROUTS				
cooked	1 lb	152	21	3
raw	½ cup	27	4	tr

KIWIFRUIT

fresh	1 med	46	11	tr

KOHLRABI

FRESH				
raw; sliced	½ cup	19	4	tr
sliced, cooked	½ cup	24	5	tr

KUMQUATS

fresh	1	12	3	tr

LAMB

FRESH				
cubed, lean only, raw	1 oz	38	0	2
cubed, lean only; braised	3 oz	190	0	7
cubed, lean only; broiled	3 oz	158	0	6
ground, raw	1 oz	80	0	7

FOOD	PORTION	CALORIES	CHO	FAT
ground; broiled	3 oz	240	0	17
leg, lean & fat, Choice; roasted	3 oz	219	14	14
loin chop w/bone lean & fat, Choice, raw	1 chop (3.3 oz)	294	0	15
loin chop w/bone lean & fat, Choice; broiled	1 chop (2.3 oz)	201	0	15
loin chop w/bone lean only, Choice; broiled	1 chop (1.6 oz)	100	0	5
rib chop, lean only, Choice; broiled	3 oz	200	0	11
rib chop, lean & fat, Choice; broiled	3 oz	307	0	25
shank, lean & fat, Choice; braised	3 oz	206	0	11
shank, lean & fat, Choice; roasted	3 oz	191	0	11
shoulder chop w/ bone, lean & fat, Choice, raw	1 chop (4.7 oz)	346	0	28
shoulder chop, w/ bone, lean only, Choice, raw	1 chop (3.5 oz)	133	0	5
shoulder chop, w/ bone, lean only, Choice; braised	1 chop (1.9 oz)	152	0	8
shoulder chop, w/ bone, lean & fat, Choice; braised	1 chop (2.5 oz)	244	0	17
sirloin, lean & fat, Choice; roasted	3 oz	248	0	21
FROZEN New Zealand, lean & fat, raw	1 oz	79	0	6

FOOD	PORTION	CALORIES	CHO	FAT
New Zealand, lean & fat; cooked	3 oz	259	0	19
New Zealand, lean only, raw	1 oz	36	0	1
New Zealand, lean only; cooked	3 oz	175	0	8

LAMBSQUARTERS

FRESH
chopped, cooked	½ cup	29	5	1

LEEKS

DRIED
freeze dried	1 tbsp	1	tr	0

FRESH
chopped, cooked	¼ cup	8	2	tr
cooked	1 (4.4 oz)	38	9	tr
raw	1 (4.4 oz)	76	18	tr
raw; chopped	¼ cup	16	4	tr

LEMON

lemon	1 med	22	12	tr
peel	1 tbsp	0	1	tr
wedge	1	5	3	tr

JUICE
bottled	1 tbsp	3	1	tr
fresh	1 tbsp	4	1	0
frzn	1 tbsp	3	1	tr

FOOD	PORTION	CALORIES	CHO	FAT
LENTILS				
DRIED				
cooked	1 cup	231	40	1
raw	1 cup	649	110	2
SPROUTS				
raw	½ cup	40	8	tr
LETTUCE				
bibb	1 head (6 oz)	21	4	tr
Boston	2 leaves	2	tr	tr
Boston	1 head (6 oz)	21	4	tr
iceberg	1 leaf	3	tr	tr
iceberg	1 head (19 oz)	70	11	1
looseleaf; shredded	½ cup	5	1	tr
romaine; shredded	½ cup	4	1	tr
LIMA BEANS				
CANNED				
large	1 cup	191	36	tr
lima beans	½ cup	93	17	tr
DRIED				
baby, raw	1 cup	677	127	2
baby; cooked	1 cup	229	42	1
cooked	½ cup	104	20	tr
large, raw	1 cup	602	113	1
large; cooked	1 cup	217	39	1

FOOD	PORTION	CALORIES	CHO	FAT
FROZEN				
cooked	½ cup	94	18	tr
fordhook; cooked	½ cup	85	16	tr
LIME				
FRESH				
lime	1	20	7	tr
JUICE				
bottled	1 tbsp	3	1	tr
fresh	1 tbsp	4	1	tr
LINCOD				
FRESH				
blue, raw	3½ oz	83	0	1
LING				
raw	3 oz	74	0	1
LINGCOD				
raw	3 oz	72	0	1
LIQUOR/LIQUEUR				
Bloody Mary	5 oz	116	5	tr
bourbon & soda	4 oz	105	0	0
*coffee liqueur	1½ oz	174	24	tr
*coffee w/ cream liqueur	1½ oz	154	10	7
*crème de menthe	1½ oz	186	21	tr
*daiquiri	2 oz	111	4	0

FOOD	PORTION	CALORIES	CHO	FAT
gin	1½ oz	110	0	0
gin & tonic	7.5 oz	171	16	0
Manhattan	2 oz	128	2	0
martini	2½ oz	156	tr	0
*piña colada	4½ oz	262	40	3
rum	1½ oz	97	0	0
screwdriver	7 oz	174	18	tr
*tequila sunrise	5½ oz	189	15	tr
*Tom Collins	7½ oz	121	3	0
vodka	1½ oz	97	0	0
whiskey	1½ oz	105	tr	0
*whiskey sour	3 oz	123	5	tr
*whiskey sour mix, not prep	1 pkg (.6 oz)	64	16	0
*whiskey sour mix; as prep	3.6 oz	169	16	0

LIVER

FOOD	PORTION	CALORIES	CHO	FAT
beef; braised	3 oz	137	3	4
beef; pan-fried	3 oz	184	7	7
chicken, raw	1 (1.1 oz)	40	1	1
chicken; stewed	1 cup (5 oz)	219	1	8
duck, raw	1 (1.5 oz)	60	2	2
goose, raw	1 (3.3 oz)	125	6	4
lamb; braised	3 oz	187	2	7
lamb; fried	3 oz	202	3	11
pork; braised	3 oz	141	3	4

FOOD	PORTION	CALORIES	CHO	FAT
sheep, raw	3½ oz	131	0	4
turkey; raw	1 (3.6 oz)	140	4	4
turkey; simmered	1 cup (5 oz)	237	5	8
veal; braised	3 oz	140	2	6
veal; fried	3 oz	208	3	10

LOBSTER

FRESH
northern, raw	3 oz	77	tr	1
northern, raw	1 lobster (5.3 oz)	136	1	1
northern; cooked	1 cup	142	2	1
northern; cooked	3 oz	83	1	1
spiny, raw	3 oz	95	2	1
spiny, raw	1 (7.3 oz)	233	5	3

LOGANBERRIES

frzn	1 cup	80	19	tr

LONGANS

fresh	1	2	tr	0

LOQUATS

fresh	1	5	1	tr

LOTUS

root, raw; sliced	10 slices	45	14	tr
root; sliced, cooked	10 slices	59	14	tr

FOOD	PORTION	CALORIES	CHO	FAT
seeds, dried	1 oz	94	18	1

LUNCHEON MEATS/COLD CUTS

FOOD	PORTION	CALORIES	CHO	FAT
barbecue loaf, pork & beef	1 oz	49	2	3
beerwurst, beef	1 slice (1/16" × 2¾")	19	tr	2
beerwurst, beef	1 slice (4" × 1/8")	75	tr	7
beerwurst, pork	1 slice (2¾" × 1/16")	14	tr	1
beerwurst, pork	1 slice (4" × 1/8")	55	tr	4
berliner, pork & beef	1 oz	65	1	4
blood sausage	1 oz	95	tr	9
bologna, beef	1 oz	72	tr	7
bologna, beef & pork	1 oz	89	1	8
bologna, pork	1 oz	70	tr	6
braunschweiger, pork	1 slice (2½" × ¼")	65	1	6
braunschweiger, pork	1 oz	102	1	9
corned beef loaf	1 oz	46	0	2
dried beef	1 oz	47	tr	1
dried beef	5 slices (21 g)	35	tr	tr
Dutch brand loaf, pork & beef	1 oz	68	2	5
headcheese, pork	1 oz	60	tr	4
honey loaf, pork & beef	1 oz	36	2	1

FOOD	PORTION	CALORIES	CHO	FAT
honey roll sausage, beef	1 oz	42	1	2
Lebanon bologna, beef	1 oz	64	1	4
liver cheese, pork	1 oz	86	1	7
liverwurst, pork	1 oz	93	1	8
luncheon meat, beef	1 oz	87	1	7
luncheon meat, pork & beef	1 oz	100	1	9
luncheon meat, pork, canned	1 oz	95	1	9
luncheon sausage pork & beef	1 oz	74	tr	6
luxury loaf, pork	1 oz	40	1	1
mortadella, beef & pork	1 oz	88	1	7
mother's loaf, pork	1 oz	80	2	6
New England brand sausage, pork & beef	1 oz	46	1	2
olive loaf, pork	1 oz	67	3	5
peppered loaf, pork & beef	1 oz	42	1	2
pepperoni, pork & beef	1 (9 oz)	1248	7	110
pepperoni, pork & beef	slice (.2 oz)	27	tr	2
pickle & pimiento loaf, pork	1 oz	74	2	6
picnic loaf, pork & beef	1 oz	66	1	5
salami, cooked, beef & pork	1 oz	71	1	6
salami, hard, pork	1 slice (⅓ oz)	41	3	4
salami, hard, pork	1 pkg (4 oz)	460	2	38
salami, hard, pork & beef	1 slice (⅓ oz)	42	tr	3
salami, hard, pork & beef	1 pkg (4 oz)	472	3	39

FOOD	PORTION	CALORIES	CHO	FAT
sandwich spread, pork & beef	1 tbsp	35	2	3
sandwich spread, pork & beef	1 oz	67	3	5
summer sausage, Thuringer, cervelat	1 oz	98	1	8
TAKE-OUT submarine w/ salami, ham, cheese, lettuce, tomato, onion, oil	1	456	51	19

LUPINES

DRIED				
cooked	1 cup	197	16	5
raw	1 cup	668	73	17

LYCHEES

fresh	1	6	2	tr

MACADAMIA NUTS

dried	1 oz	199	4	21
oil roasted	1 oz	204	4	22

MACE

ground	1 tsp	8	1	1

MACKEREL

CANNED				
jack	1 can (12.7 oz)	563	0	23

FOOD	PORTION	CALORIES	CHO	FAT
jack	1 cup	296	0	12
FRESH				
Atlantic, raw	3 oz	174	0	12
Atlantic; cooked	3 oz	223	0	15
king, raw	3 oz	89	0	2
Spanish, raw	3 oz	118	0	5
Spanish; cooked	1 fillet (5.1 oz)	230	0	9
Spanish; cooked	3 oz	134	0	5

MALT

malt beverage nonalcoholic	12 oz	32	5	0

MALTED MILK

POWDER				
*chocolate	3 heaping tsp (¾ oz)	83	18	1
*natural flavor	3 heaping tsp (¾ oz)	86	15	2
PREPARED				
*chocolate; as prep w/ whole milk	1 cup	233	29	9
*natural flavor; as prep w/ whole milk	1 cup	236	27	10

MAMMY APPLE

fresh	1	431	106	4

FOOD	PORTION	CALORIES	CHO	FAT
MANGO				
fresh	1	135	35	1
MARGARINE				
REDUCED CALORIE				
diet	1 tsp	17	0	2
diet	1 cup	800	1	90
REGULAR				
corn	1 stick (4 oz)	815	1	91
corn	1 tsp	34	0	4
salted	1 stick (4 oz)	815	1	91
salted	1 tsp	39	0	4
unsalted	1 stick (4 oz)	809	1	91
unsalted	1 tsp	34	0	4
SOFT				
corn	1 tsp	34	0	4
corn	1 cup	1626	1	183
safflower	1 tsp	34	0	4
safflower	1 cup	1626	1	183
soybean, salted	1 tsp	34	0	4
soybean, salted	1 cup	1626	1	183
soybean, unsalted	1 cup	1626	2	182
soybean, unsalted	1 tsp	34	0	4
tub, salted	1 cup	1626	1	183
tub, salted	1 tsp	34	0	4
tub, unsalted	1 cup	1626	0	182

FOOD	PORTION	CALORIES	CHO	FAT
tub, unsalted	1 tsp	34	0	4
SQUEEZE				
soybean & cottonseed	1 tsp	34	0	4

MARJORAM

dried	1 tsp	2	tr	tr

MAYONNAISE

REDUCED CALORIE				
reduced calorie	1 tbsp	34	2	3
reduced calorie	1 cup	556	38	46
REGULAR				
mayonnaise	1 tbsp	99	tr	11
mayonnaise	1 cup	1577	6	175
sandwich spread	1 tbsp	60	3	5

MAYONNAISE TYPE SALAD DRESSING

REDUCED CALORIE				
reduced calorie w/o cholesterol	1 cup	1084	36	107
reduced calorie w/o cholesterol	1 tbsp	68	2	7
REGULAR				
home recipe	1 tbsp	25	2	2
home recipe	1 cup	400	38	24
mayonnaise type salad dressing	1 cup	916	56	78
mayonnaise type salad dressing	1 tbsp	57	4	5

FOOD	PORTION	CALORIES	CHO	FAT
MEAT SUBSTITUTES				
simulated sausage	1 link (25 g)	64	2	5
simulated sausage	1 patty (38 g)	97	4	7
MELON				
FROZEN				
melon balls	1 cup	55	14	tr
MEXICAN FOOD				
CANNED				
refried beans	½ cup	134	23	1
READY-TO-USE				
tortilla, corn	1 (1 oz)	65	13	1
TAKE-OUT				
*burrito w/ apple	1 sm (2.6 oz)	231	35	10
*burrito w/ apple	1 lg (5.4 oz)	484	73	20
*burrito w/ cherry	1 sm (2.6 oz)	231	35	10
*burrito w/ cherry	1 lg (5.4 oz)	484	73	20
burrito w/ beans	2 (7.6 oz)	448	71	14
burrito w/ beans & cheese	2 (6.5 oz)	377	55	12
burrito w/ beans & chili peppers	2 (7.2 oz)	413	58	15
burrito w/ beans & meat	2 (8.1 oz)	508	66	18
burrito w/ beef	2 (7.7 oz)	523	59	21
burrito w/ beef & chili peppers	2 (7.1 oz)	426	49	17
burrito w/ beef, cheese & chili peppers	2 (10.7 oz)	634	64	25

FOOD	PORTION	CALORIES	CHO	FAT
burrito w/ beans, cheese & beef	2 (7.1 oz)	331	40	13
burrito w/ beans, cheese & chili peppers	2 (11.8 oz)	663	85	23
chimichanga w/ beef	1 (6.1 oz)	425	43	20
chimichanga w/ beef & cheese	1 (6.4 oz)	443	39	23
chimichanga w/ beef & red chili peppers	1 (6.7 oz)	424	46	19
chimichanga w/ beef, cheese & red chili peppers	1 (6.3 oz)	364	38	18
enchilada w/ cheese	1 (5.7 oz)	320	29	19
enchilada w/ cheese & beef	1 (6.7 oz)	324	30	18
enchirito w/ cheese, beef & beans	1 (6.8 oz)	344	34	16
frijoles w/ cheese	1 cup (5.9 oz)	226	29	8
nachos w/ cheese	6 to 8 (4 oz)	345	36	19
nachos w/ cheese & jalapeno peppers	6 to 8 (7.2 oz)	607	60	34
nachos w/ cheese, beans, ground beef & peppers	6 to 8 (8.9 oz)	568	56	31
*nachos w/ cinnamon & sugar	6 to 8 (3.8 oz)	592	63	36
taco	1 sm (6 oz)	370	27	21
taco salad	1½ cups	279	24	15
taco salad w/ chili con carne	1½ cups	288	27	13
tostada w/ beans & cheese	1 (5.1 oz)	223	27	10

FOOD	PORTION	CALORIES	CHO	FAT
tostada w/ beans, beef & cheese	1 (7.9 oz)	334	30	17
tostada w/ beef & cheese	1 (5.7 oz)	315	23	16
tostada w/ guacamole	2 (9.2 oz)	360	32	23

MILK

CANNED

FOOD	PORTION	CALORIES	CHO	FAT
*condensed, sweetened	1 oz	123	21	3
*condensed, sweetened	1 cup	982	166	27
evaporated	½ cup	169	13	10
evaporated, skim	½ cup	99	14	tr
DRIED				
buttermilk	1 tbsp	25	3	tr
nonfat, instant	1 pkg (3.2 oz)	244	47	tr
LIQUID, LOWFAT				
1%, protein fortified	1 cup	119	14	3
1%	1 cup	102	12	3
1%	1 qt	409	47	10
1%, protein fortified	1 qt	476	54	12
2%	1 cup	121	12	5
2%	1 qt	485	47	19
buttermilk	1 cup	99	12	2
buttermilk	1 qt	396	47	9
LIQUID, REGULAR				
buffalo milk	3½ oz	112	5	8
camel milk	3½ oz	80	5	4

FOOD	PORTION	CALORIES	CHO	FAT
donkey milk	3½ oz	43	6	1
goat milk	1 cup	168	11	10
goat milk	1 qt	672	43	40
human milk	1 cup	171	17	11
Indian buffalo milk	1 cup	236	13	17
low sodium	1 cup	149	11	8
mare milk	3½ oz	49	6	2
sheep milk	1 cup	264	13	17
whole	1 cup	150	11	8
LIQUID, SKIM				
skim	1 cup	86	12	tr
skim	1 qt	342	48	2
skim, protein fortified	1 cup	100	14	1
skim, protein fortified	1 qt	400	55	2

MILK DRINKS

FOOD	PORTION	CALORIES	CHO	FAT
*chocolate milk	1 cup	208	26	8
*chocolate milk	1 qt	833	103	34
*chocolate milk, 1% fat	1 cup	158	26	3
*chocolate milk, 1% fat	1 qt	630	104	10
*chocolate milk, 2% fat	1 cup	179	26	5
*strawberry flavor mix; as prep w/ whole milk	9 oz	234	33	8

MILK SUBSTITUTES

FOOD	PORTION	CALORIES	CHO	FAT
imitation milk	1 cup	150	15	8
imitation milk	1 qt	600	60	33

FOOD	PORTION	CALORIES	CHO	FAT
MILKFISH				
FRESH				
raw	3 oz	126	0	6
MILKSHAKE				
*chocolate	10 oz	360	58	11
*chocolate thick shake	10.6 oz	356	63	8
*strawberry	10 oz	319	53	8
*vanilla	10 oz	314	51	8
*vanilla thick shake	11 oz	350	56	10
MILLET				
cooked	½ cup	143	28	1
raw	½ cup	378	73	4
MISO				
miso	½ cup	284	39	8
MOLASSES				
*blackstrap	2 tbsp	85	22	0
*molasses	2 tbsp	85	22	0
MONKFISH				
FRESH				
raw	3 oz	64	0	1
MOOSE				
raw	1 oz	29	0	tr
roasted	3 oz	114	0	1

FOOD	PORTION	CALORIES	CHO	FAT
MOTH BEANS				
DRIED				
cooked	1 cup	207	37	1
raw	1 cup	673	121	3
MUFFIN				
HOME RECIPE				
*blueberry	1 (1.5 oz)	135	20	5
*bran	1 (1.5 oz)	125	19	6
MIX				
*blueberry	1 (1.5 oz)	140	22	5
*bran	1 (1.5 oz)	140	24	4
*corn	1 (1.5 oz)	145	22	6
MULBERRIES				
fresh	1 cup	61	14	1
MULLET				
FRESH				
striped, raw	3 oz	99	0	3
striped; cooked	3 oz	127	0	4
MUNG BEANS				
DRIED				
cooked	1 cup	213	39	1
raw	1 cup	719	130	2
SPROUTS				
canned	½ cup	8	1	

FOOD	PORTION	CALORIES	CHO	FAT
cooked	½ cup	13	3	tr
raw	½ cup	16	3	tr
stir fried	½ cup	31	7	tr

MUNGO BEANS

DRIED
cooked	1 cup	190	33	1
raw	1 cup	726	126	4

MUSHROOMS

CANNED
chanterelle	3½ oz	12	tr	1
pieces	½ cup	19	4	tr
whole	1 (.4 oz)	3	1	tr

DRIED
chanterelle	3½ oz	89	2	2
shiitake	4 (½ oz)	44	11	tr

FRESH
chanterelle	3½ oz	11	tr	tr
morel	3½ oz	9	0	tr
raw	1 (½ oz)	5	1	tr
raw; sliced	½ cup	9	2	tr
shiitake; cooked	4 (2.5 oz)	40	10	tr
sliced, cooked	½ cup	21	4	tr
whole; cooked	1 (.4 oz)	3	1	tr

FOOD	PORTION	CALORIES	CHO	FAT
MUSKRAT				
raw	1 oz	46	0	2
roasted	3 oz	156	0	8
MUSSELS				
FRESH				
blue, raw	3 oz	73	3	2
blue, raw	1 cup	129	6	3
blue; cooked	3 oz	147	6	4
MUSTARD				
yellow	1 tsp	5	tr	tr
DRY				
mustard seed, yellow	1 tsp	15	1	1
MUSTARD GREENS				
FRESH				
chopped, cooked	½ cup	11	1	tr
raw; chopped	½ cup	7	1	tr
FROZEN				
chopped; cooked	½ cup	14	2	tr
NATTO				
natto	½ cup	187	13	10
NAVY BEANS				
CANNED				
navy	1 cup	296	54	1

FOOD	PORTION	CALORIES	CHO	FAT
DRIED				
cooked	1 cup	259	48	1
raw	1 cup	697	126	3
SPROUTS				
cooked	3½ oz	78	15	1
raw	½ cup	35	8	tr

NECTARINE

fresh	1	67	16	1

NOODLES

DRY				
cellophane	1 cup	492	121	tr
chow mein	1 cup	237	26	14
egg	½ cup	145	27	2
egg; cooked	1 cup	212	40	2
Japanese soba	2 oz	192	43	tr
Japanese soba; cooked	½ cup	56	12	tr
Japanese somen	2 oz	203	42	tr
Japanese somen; cooked	½ cup	115	24	tr
spinach/egg	1 cup	145	27	2
spinach/egg; cooked	1 cup	211	39	3

NUTMEG

ground	1 tsp	12	1	1

NUTS, MIXED

dry roasted w/ peanuts	1 oz	169	7	15

FOOD	PORTION	CALORIES	CHO	FAT
dry roasted w/ peanuts, salted	1 oz	169	7	15
oil roasted w/ peanuts	1 oz	175	6	16
oil roasted w/ peanuts, salted	1 oz	175	6	16
oil roasted w/o peanuts	1 oz	175	6	16
oil roasted w/o peanuts, salted	1 oz	175	6	16

OCTOPUS

FRESH
raw	3 oz	70	2	1

OHELOBERRIES

fresh	1 cup	39	10	tr

OIL

almond	1 cup	1927	0	218
almond	1 tbsp	120	0	14
apricot kernel	1 cup	1927	0	218
apricot kernel	1 tbsp	120	0	14
canola	1 tbsp	120	0	14
canola	1 cup	1927	0	218
coconut	1 tbsp	120	0	14
corn	1 cup	1927	0	218
corn	1 tbsp	120	0	14
cottonseed	1 cup	1927	0	218

FOOD	PORTION	CALORIES	CHO	FAT
cottonseed	1 tbsp	120	0	14
cupu assu	1 tbsp	120	0	14
grapeseed	1 tbsp	120	0	14
hazelnut	1 cup	1927	0	218
hazelnut	1 tbsp	120	0	14
herring	3½ oz	945	0	100
olive	1 tbsp	119	0	14
olive	1 cup	1909	0	216
palm	1 cup	1927	0	218
palm	1 tbsp	120	0	14
palm kernel	1 tbsp	120	0	14
palm kernel	1 cup	1927	0	218
palm, babassu	1 tbsp	120	0	14
peanut	1 cup	1909	0	216
peanut	1 tbsp	119	0	14
poppyseed	1 tbsp	120	0	14
pumpkin seed	3½ oz	925	0	100
rice bran	1 tbsp	120	0	14
safflower	1 tbsp	120	0	14
safflower	1 cup	1927	0	218
sesame	1 tbsp	120	0	14
shark	3½ oz	945	0	100
sheanut	1 tbsp	120	0	14
soybean	1 tbsp	120	0	14
soybean	1 cup	1927	0	218

FOOD	PORTION	CALORIES	CHO	FAT
sunflower	1 tbsp	120	0	14
sunflower	1 cup	1927	0	218
teaseed	1 tbsp	120	0	14
tomatoseed	1 tbsp	120	0	14
vegetable, soybean & cottonseed	1 tbsp	120	0	14
vegetable, soybean & cottonseed	1 cup	1927	0	218
walnut	1 cup	1927	0	218
walnut	1 tbsp	120	0	14
whale	3½ oz	945	0	100
wheat germ	1 tbsp	120	0	14

OKRA

FRESH
raw	8 pods	36	7	tr
raw; sliced	½ cup	19	4	tr
sliced, cooked	½ cup	25	6	tr
sliced, cooked	8 pods	27	6	tr

FROZEN
| sliced; cooked | ½ cup | 34 | 8 | tr |
| sliced; cooked | 1 pkg (10 oz) | 94 | 21 | 1 |

OLIVES

| green | 4 med | 15 | tr | 2 |
| green | 3 extra lg | 15 | tr | 2 |

FOOD	PORTION	CALORIES	CHO	FAT
ripe	3 sm	15	tr	2
ripe	2 lg	15	tr	2

ONION

FOOD	PORTION	CALORIES	CHO	FAT
CANNED				
chopped	½ cup	21	5	tr
whole	1 (2.2 oz)	12	3	tr
DRIED				
flakes	1 tbsp	16	4	tr
powder	1 tsp	7	2	tr
FRESH				
chopped, cooked	½ cup	29	7	tr
raw; chopped	1 tbsp	3	1	tr
raw; chopped	½ cup	27	6	tr
scallions, raw; chopped	1 tbsp	2	tr	tr
scallions, raw; sliced	½ cup	13	3	tr
Welsh, raw	3½ oz	34	7	tr
FROZEN				
chopped; cooked	1 tbsp	4	1	tr
chopped; cooked	½ cup	30	7	tr
rings	7 (2.5 oz)	285	27	19
rings; cooked	2 (.7 oz)	81	8	5
whole; cooked	3½ oz	28	7	tr
TAKE-OUT				
rings: breaded & fried	8 to 9	275	31	16

FOOD	PORTION	CALORIES	CHO	FAT
OPOSSUM				
roasted	3 oz	188	0	9
ORANGE				
FRESH				
California Valencia	1	59	14	tr
California navel	1	65	16	tr
Florida	1	69	17	tr
peel	1 tbsp	6	2	tr
sections	1 cup	85	21	tr
JUICE				
canned	1 cup	104	25	tr
chilled	1 cup	110	25	1
fresh	1 cup	111	26	tr
frzn, not prep	6 oz	339	81	tr
frzn; as prep	1 cup	112	27	tr
mandarin orange	3½ oz	47	10	tr
*orange drink	6 oz	94	24	0
OREGANO				
ground	1 tsp	5	1	tr
ORIENTAL FOOD				
CANNED				
chow mein chicken	1 cup	95	18	tr
HOME RECIPE				
chop suey w/ beef & pork	1 cup	300	13	17
chow mein chicken	1 cup	255	10	10

FOOD	PORTION	CALORIES	CHO	FAT

OYSTERS

CANNED

FOOD	PORTION	CALORIES	CHO	FAT
eastern	1 cup	170	10	6
eastern	3 oz	58	3	2

FRESH

FOOD	PORTION	CALORIES	CHO	FAT
eastern, raw	6 med	58	3	2
eastern, raw	1 cup	170	10	6
eastern; cooked	6 med	58	3	2
eastern; cooked	3 oz	117	7	4
Pacific, raw	3 oz	69	4	2
Pacific, raw	1 med	41	2	1

HOME RECIPE

FOOD	PORTION	CALORIES	CHO	FAT
eastern; breaded & fried	3 oz	167	10	11
eastern; breaded & fried	6 medium	173	10	11

TAKE-OUT

FOOD	PORTION	CALORIES	CHO	FAT
battered & fried	6 (4.9 oz)	368	40	18
breaded & fried	6 (4.9 oz)	368	40	18

PANCAKES

HOME RECIPE

FOOD	PORTION	CALORIES	CHO	FAT
plain	1 (4" diam)	60	9	2

MIX

FOOD	PORTION	CALORIES	CHO	FAT
buckwheat	1 (4" diam)	55	6	2

TAKE-OUT

FOOD	PORTION	CALORIES	CHO	FAT
*w/ butter & syrup	3	519	91	14

PANCAKE/WAFFLE SYRUP

FOOD	PORTION	CALORIES	CHO	FAT
low calorie	1 tbsp	12	3	0

FOOD	PORTION	CALORIES	CHO	FAT
*maple	2 tbsp	122	32	0

PAPAYA

FRESH				
cubed	1 cup	54	14	tr
papaya	1	117	30	tr
JUICE				
nectar	1 cup	142	36	tr

PAPRIKA

paprika	1 tsp	6	1	tr

PARSLEY

dried	1 tsp	1	tr	tr
dried	1 tbsp	1	tr	tr
fresh, raw; chopped	½ cup	10	2	tr

PARSNIPS

FRESH				
cooked	1 (5.6 oz)	130	31	tr
cooked, sliced	½ cup	63	15	tr
raw; sliced	½ cup	50	12	tr

PASSION FRUIT

purple	1	18	4	tr
JUICE				
purple	1 cup	126	34	tr
yellow	1 cup	149	36	tr

FOOD	PORTION	CALORIES	CHO	FAT

PASTA

DRY

FOOD	PORTION	CALORIES	CHO	FAT
corn	2 oz	204	45	1
corn; cooked	1 cup	176	39	1
elbows	1 cup	389	78	2
elbows; cooked	1 cup	197	40	tr
protein-fortified	1 cup	348	63	2
protein-fortified; cooked	1 cup	188	36	tr
shells	1 cup	389	78	2
shells; cooked	1 cup	197	40	tr
spaghetti	2 oz	211	43	tr
spaghetti, protein fortified	2 oz	214	39	1
spaghetti, protein fortified; cooked	1 cup	229	44	tr
spaghetti; cooked	1 cup	197	40	tr
spinach spaghetti	2 oz	212	43	tr
spinach spaghetti; cooked	1 cup	183	37	tr
spirals	1 cup	389	78	2
spirals; cooked	1 cup	197	40	tr
vegetable	1 cup	308	63	tr
vegetable; cooked	1 cup	171	36	tr
whole wheat	1 cup	365	79	1
whole wheat spaghetti	2 oz	198	43	tr
whole wheat spaghetti; cooked	1 cup	174	37	tr
whole wheat; cooked	1 cup	174	37	tr

FOOD	PORTION	CALORIES	CHO	FAT
FRESH				
plain made w/ egg	4.5 oz	368	70	3
plain made w/ egg; cooked	2 oz	75	14	tr
spinach made w/ egg	4.5 oz	370	71	3
spinach made w/ egg; cooked	2 oz	74	14	tr
HOME RECIPE				
made w/ egg; cooked	2 oz	74	13	tr

PASTA DINNERS

CANNED				
macaroni & cheese	1 cup	230	26	10
HOME RECIPE				
macaroni & cheese	1 cup	430	40	22
spaghetti w/ meatballs & tomato sauce	1 cup	330	39	12

PÂTÉ

CANNED				
chicken liver	1 tbsp	109	1	2
chicken liver	1 oz	238	2	4
goose liver, smoked	1 tbsp	60	1	6
goose liver, smoked*	1 oz	131	1	12
liver	1 tbsp	41	tr	4
liver	1 oz	90	tr	8

PEACH

*halves in heavy syrup	1 half	60	16	tr
*halves in light syrup	1 half	44	12	tr

FOOD	PORTION	CALORIES	CHO	FAT
halves, juice pack	1 half	34	9	tr
halves, juice pack	1 half	38	10	tr
halves, water pack	1 half	18	5	tr
*spiced in heavy syrup	1 fruit	66	18	tr
*spiced in heavy syrup	1 cup	180	49	tr
DRIED				
halves	10	311	80	1
halves	1 cup	383	98	1
*halves; cooked w/ sugar	½ cup	139	36	tr
halves; cooked w/o sugar	½ cup	99	25	tr
FRESH				
peach	1	37	10	tr
sliced	1 cup	73	19	tr
FROZEN				
*slices, sweetened	1 cup	235	60	tr
JUICE				
nectar	1 cup	134	35	tr

PEANUT BUTTER

*chunk style	1 cup	1520	56	129
*chunk style	2 tbsp	188	7	16
*smooth	1 tbsp	95	3	8
*smooth	1 cup	1526	41	132
*smooth w/o salt	1 tbsp	95	3	8
*smooth w/o salt	1 cup	1526	41	132

FOOD	PORTION	CALORIES	CHO	FAT
PEANUTS				
boiled	½ cup	102	7	7
dried	1 oz	161	5	14
dry roasted	1 cup	855	31	73
dry roasted	1 oz	164	6	14
oil roasted	1 oz	165	5	14
oil roasted	1 cup	841	27	71
Spanish, oil roasted	1 oz	162	5	14
Spanish, oil roasted	1 cup	851	26	72
Valencia, oil roasted	1 cup	848	23	74
Valencia, oil roasted	1 oz	165	5	14
Virginia, oil roasted	1 oz	161	5	14
Virginia, oil roasted	1 cup	826	28	70
PEAR				
CANNED				
*halves in heavy syrup	1 cup	188	49	tr
*halves in heavy syrup	1 half	68	15	tr
*halves in light syrup	1 half	45	12	tr
halves, juice pack	1 cup	123	32	tr
halves, water pack	1 half	22	6	tr
DRIED				
halves	10	459	122	1
halves	1 cup	472	125	1

FOOD	PORTION	CALORIES	CHO	FAT
*halves; cooked w/ sugar	½ cup	196	52	tr
halves; cooked w/o sugar	½ cup	163	43	tr
FRESH				
pear	1	98	25	1
JUICE				
nectar	1 cup	149	39	tr

PEAS

CANNED				
green	½ cup	59	11	tr
DRIED				
split, raw	1 cup	671	119	2
split; cooked	1 cup	231	41	1
FRESH				
edible-pod, raw	½ cup	30	5	tr
edible-pod; cooked	½ cup	34	6	tr
green, raw	½ cup	63	11	tr
green; cooked	½ cup	67	13	tr
FROZEN				
edible-pod; cooked	1 pkg (10 oz)	132	23	1
edible-pod; cooked	½ cup	42	7	tr
green; cooked	½ cup	63	11	tr
SPROUTS				
raw	½ cup	77	17	tr

FOOD	PORTION	CALORIES	CHO	FAT

PECANS

FOOD	PORTION	CALORIES	CHO	FAT
dried	1 oz	190	5	19
dry roasted	1 oz	187	6	18
dry roasted, salted	1 oz	187	6	18
halves, dried	1 cup	721	20	73
oil roasted	1 oz	195	5	20
oil roasted, salted	1 oz	195	5	20

PEPPER

FOOD	PORTION	CALORIES	CHO	FAT
black	1 tsp	5	1	tr
cayenne	1 tsp	6	1	tr
red	1 tsp	6	1	tr
white	1 tsp	7	2	tr

PEPPERS

CANNED

FOOD	PORTION	CALORIES	CHO	FAT
chili, green, hot	1 (2.6 oz)	18	4	tr
chili, green, hot, raw	1	18	4	tr
chili, green, hot; chopped	½ cup	17	4	tr
chili, red, hot	1 (2.6 oz)	18	4	tr
chili, red, hot; chopped	½ cup	17	4	tr
green, halves	½ cup	13	3	tr
jalapeno; chopped	½ cup	17	3	tr
red, halves	½ cup	13	3	tr

DRIED

FOOD	PORTION	CALORIES	CHO	FAT
green	1 tbsp	1	tr	tr

FOOD	PORTION	CALORIES	CHO	FAT
red	1 tbsp	1	tr	tr
FRESH				
chili, green, hot, raw; chopped	½ cup	30	7	tr
chili, red, hot, raw	1 (1.6 oz)	18	4	tr
chili, red, raw; chopped	½ cup	30	7	tr
green, raw	1 (2.6 oz)	18	4	tr
green; cooked	1 (2.6 oz)	13	3	tr
green; cooked	½ cup	13	3	tr
red, raw	1 (2.6 oz)	18	4	tr
red; chopped, cooked	½ cup	12	3	tr
red; cooked	1 (2.6 oz)	13	3	tr
FROZEN				
green, chopped; not prep	1 oz	6	1	tr
red, chopped; not prep	1 oz	6	1	tr

PERCH

FOOD	PORTION	CALORIES	CHO	FAT
FRESH				
cooked	1 fillet (1.6 oz)	54	0	1
cooked	3 oz	99	0	1
ocean perch, Atlantic, raw	3 oz	80	0	1
ocean perch, Atlantic; cooked	1 fillet (1.8 oz)	60	0	1
ocean perch, Atlantic; cooked	3 oz	103	0	2
raw	3 oz	77	0	1
red, raw	3½ oz	114	0	4

FOOD	PORTION	CALORIES	CHO	FAT
PERSIMMONS				
dried, Japanese	1	93	25	tr
fresh	1	32	8	tr
fresh, Japanese	1	118	31	tr
PHEASANT				
FRESH				
breast w/o skin, raw	½ breast (6.4 oz)	243	0	6
leg w/o skin, raw	1 (3.6 oz)	143	0	5
w/ skin, raw	½ pheasant (14 oz)	723	0	37
w/o skin, raw	½ pheasant (12.4 oz)	470	0	13
PICKLES				
dill	1 (2.3 oz)	5	1	tr
gherkins	3½ oz	21	4	tr
quick sour; sliced	½ oz	10	3	tr
sweet gherkin	1 sm (½ oz)	20	5	tr
PIE				
CANNED FILLING				
pumpkin pie mix	1 cup	282	36	tr
HOME RECIPE				
*pecan	⅙ of 9" pie	575	71	19
READY-TO-USE				
*apple	⅙ of 9" pie	405	60	18

FOOD	PORTION	CALORIES	CHO	FAT
*blueberry	⅙ of 9" pie	380	55	17
*cherry	⅙ of 9" pie	410	61	18
*creme	⅙ of 9" pie	455	59	23
*custard	⅙ of 9" pie	330	36	17
*lemon meringue	⅙ of 9" pie	355	53	14
*peach	⅙ of 9" pie	405	60	17
*pumpkin	⅙ of 9" pie	320	37	17
SNACK				
*apple	1 (3 oz)	266	33	14
*cherry	1 (3 oz)	266	33	14
*lemon	1 (3 oz)	266	33	14

PIE CRUST

HOME RECIPE				
9-inch crust	1	900	79	60
MIX				
as prep	2 crusts	1485	141	93

PIG'S EARS AND FEET

ears, frzn; simmered	1 ear (3.7 oz)	183	0	12
feet, pickled	1 oz	58	tr	5
feet, pickled	1 lb	923	tr	73
feet; simmered	2.5 oz	138	0	9

PIGEON PEAS

DRIED				
cooked	½ cup	86	15	1

FOOD	PORTION	CALORIES	CHO	FAT
cooked	1 cup	204	39	1
raw	1 cup	704	129	3

PIKE

FRESH
northern, raw	3 oz	75	0	1
northern; cooked	½ fillet (5.4 oz)	176	0	1
northern; cooked	3 oz	96	0	1
walleye red, raw	3 oz	79	0	1

PILLNUTS

pillnuts-canarytree, dried	1 oz	204	1	23

PINE NUTS

pignolia, dried	1 oz	146	4	14
pignolia, dried	1 tbsp	51	1	5
piñon, dried	1 oz	161	5	17

PINEAPPLE

CANNED
*chunks in heavy syrup	1 cup	199	52	tr
chunks, juice pack	1 cup	150	39	tr
*crushed in heavy syrup	1 cup	199	52	tr
*slices in heavy syrup	1 slice	45	12	tr
*slices in light syrup	1 slice	30	8	tr
slices, juice pack	1 slice	35	9	tr

FOOD	PORTION	CALORIES	CHO	FAT
slices, water pack	1 slice	19	5	tr
*tidbits in heavy syrup	1 cup	199	52	tr
tidbits in juice	1 cup	150	19	tr
tidbits in water	1 cup	79	20	tr
FRESH pineapple; diced	1 cup	77	19	tr
slice	1 slice	42	10	tr
FROZEN *chunks sweetened	½ cup	104	27	tr
JUICE canned	1 cup	139	34	tr
frzn; not prep	6 oz	387	96	tr
frzn; as prep	1 cup	129	32	tr

PINK BEANS

FOOD	PORTION	CALORIES	CHO	FAT
DRIED cooked	1 cup	252	47	1
raw	1 cup	721	135	2

PINTO BEANS

FOOD	PORTION	CALORIES	CHO	FAT
CANNED pinto	1 cup	186	35	1
DRIED cooked	1 cup	235	44	1
raw	1 cup	656	122	2
FROZEN cooked	3 oz	152	29	tr

FOOD	PORTION	CALORIES	CHO	FAT
SPROUTS				
cooked	3½ oz	22	4	tr
raw	3½ oz	62	12	1
PISTACHIOS				
dried	1 oz	164	7	14
dried	1 cup	739	32	62
dry roasted	1 oz	172	8	15
dry roasted, salted	1 oz	172	8	15
dry roasted, salted	1 cup	776	35	68
PITANGA				
fresh	1	2	1	tr
fresh	1 cup	57	13	1
PIZZA				
TAKE-OUT				
cheese	⅛ of 12″ pie	109	16	3
cheese	12″ pie	873	128	20
cheese, meat & vegetables	⅛ of 12″ pie	152	18	4
cheese, meat & vegetables	12″ pie	1213	140	35
pepperoni	⅛ of 12″ pie	135	15	5
pepperoni	12″ pie	1081	119	42
PLANTAINS				
FRESH				
sliced; cooked	½ cup	89	24	tr
uncooked	1	218	57	1

FOOD	PORTION	CALORIES	CHO	FAT
PLUMS				
CANNED				
*purple in heavy syrup	3	119	31	tr
*purple in heavy syrup	1 cup	320	60	tr
*purple in light syrup	3	83	22	tr
*purple in light syrup	1 cup	158	41	tr
purple, juice pack	3	55	14	tr
purple, juice pack	1 cup	146	38	tr
purple, water pack	3	39	10	tr
purple, water pack	1 cup	102	27	tr
FRESH				
plum	1	36	9	tr
sliced	1 cup	91	21	1
POI				
poi	½ cup	134	33	tr
POKEBERRY SHOOTS				
FRESH				
cooked	½ cup	16	3	tr
raw	½ cup	18	3	tr
POLLOCK				
Atlantic, raw	3 oz	78	0	1
walleye, raw	3 oz	68	0	1
walleye; cooked	1 fillet (2.1 oz)	68	0	1
walleye; cooked	3 oz	96	0	1

OOD	PORTION	CALORIES	CHO	FAT
POMEGRANATES				
pomegranates	1	104	26	tr
POMPANO				
Florida, raw	3 oz	140	0	8
Florida; cooked	3 oz	179	0	10
POPCORN				
air-popped	1 cup	30	6	tr
popped w/ vegetable oil	1 cup	55	6	3
sugar syrup coated	1 cup	135	30	1
POPPY SEEDS				
poppy seeds	1 tsp	15	1	1
PORK				
FRESH				
blade chop; roasted	1 (3.1 oz)	321	0	27
center loin chop; broiled	1 (3.1 oz)	275	0	24
center loin; roasted	3 oz	259	0	18
loin w/ fat; roasted	3 oz	271	0	21
shoulder, whole; roasted	3 oz	277	0	22
spareribs; braised	3 oz	338	0	26
tenderloin, lean only; roasted	3 oz	141	0	4

FOOD	PORTION	CALORIES	CHO	FAT

POT PIE

HOME RECIPE

beef; baked	⅓ of 9" pie (7.4 oz)	515	39	30
chicken	⅓ of 9" pie (8.1 oz)	545	42	31

POTATO

CANNED

potatoes	½ cup	54	12	tr

FRESH

baked w/ skin	1 (6½ oz)	220	51	tr
baked w/o skin	1 (5 oz)	145	34	tr
baked w/o skin	½ cup	57	13	tr
baked, skin only	1 skin (2 oz)	115	27	tr
boiled	½ cup	68	16	tr
microwaved	1 (7 oz)	212	49	tr
microwaved w/o skin	½ cup	78	18	tr
raw w/o skin	1 (3.9 oz)	88	20	tr

FROZEN

French fries, thick cut; as prep	10 strips	109	17	4
French fries; as prep	10 strips	111	17	4
hash brown; as prep	½ cup	170	22	9
potato puffs, as prep	½ cup	138	19	7
potato puffs; as prep	1 puff	16	2	<

HOME RECIPE

au gratin	½ cup	160	14	9

FOOD	PORTION	CALORIES	CHO	FAT
hash brown	½ cup	163	17	11
mashed	½ cup	111	18	4
O'Brien	1 cup	157	30	3
potato dumpling	3½ oz	334	74	1
potato pancakes	1 (2.7 oz)	495	26	13
scalloped	½ cup	105	13	5
MIX				
au gratin; as prep	4½ oz	127	18	6
instant mashed flakes; as prep	½ cup	118	16	6
instant mashed granules; as prep	½ cup	137	18	7
instant mashed granules; not prep	½ cup	80	18	tr
scalloped; as prep	4½ oz	127	18	6
TAKE-OUT				
baked, topped w/ cheese sauce	1	475	47	29
baked, topped w/ cheese sauce, bacon	1	451	44	26
baked, topped w/ cheese sauce, broccoli	1	402	47	14
baked, topped w/ cheese sauce, chili	1	481	56	22
baked, topped w/ sour cream, chives	1	394	50	22
French fried; as prep in vegetable oil	1 reg	235	29	12

FOOD	PORTION	CALORIES	CHO	FAT
French fried; as prep in vegetable oil	1 lg	355	44	19
French fried; as prep in beef tallow	1 reg	237	29	12
French fried; as prep in beef tallow	1 lg	358	44	19
hash brown	½ cup	151	16	9
mashed w/ whole milk, margarine	⅓ cup	66	13	tr
salad	½ cup	179	14	10
salad	⅓ cup	108	13	6

POTATO STARCH

potato starch	3½ oz	355	83	tr

POUT

FRESH

ocean, raw	3 oz	67	0	1

PRETZELS

sticks	10	10	2	tr
twist	1 (½ oz)	65	13	1
twists, thin	10 (2 oz)	240	48	2

PRICKLY PEAR

fresh	1	42	10	1

FOOD	PORTION	CALORIES	CHO	FAT
PRUNES				
CANNED				
*in heavy syrup	5	90	24	tr
*in heavy syrup	1 cup	245	65	tr
DRIED				
*cooked w/ sugar	½ cup	147	39	tr
cooked w/o sugar	½ cup	113	30	tr
dried	10	201	53	tr
dried	1 cup	385	101	1
JUICE				
canned	1 cup	181	45	tr
PUDDING				
HOME RECIPE				
*corn	⅔ cup	181	21	9
MIX W/ WHOLE MILK				
*chocolate, instant	½ cup	155	27	4
*chocolate, regular	½ cup	150	25	4
*rice	½ cup	155	27	4
*tapioca	½ cup	145	25	4
*vanilla, instant	½ cup	150	27	4
*vanilla, regular	½ cup	145	25	4
PUMMELO				
fresh	1	228	59	tr
sections	1 cup	71	18	tr

FOOD	PORTION	CALORIES	CHO	FAT

PUMPKIN

CANNED

FOOD	PORTION	CALORIES	CHO	FAT
pumpkin	½ cup	41	10	tr

FRESH

FOOD	PORTION	CALORIES	CHO	FAT
cooked, mashed	½ cup	24	10	tr
flowers, raw	1	0	tr	0
flowers; cooked	½ cup	10	2	tr
leaves, raw	½ cup	4	tr	tr
leaves; cooked	½ cup	7	1	tr
raw; cubed	½ cup	15	4	tr

SEEDS

FOOD	PORTION	CALORIES	CHO	FAT
roasted	1 cup	1184	31	96
roasted	1 oz	148	4	12
salted & roasted	1 cup	1184	31	96
salted & roasted	1 oz	148	4	12
seeds, dried	1 oz	154	5	13
whole, salted; roasted	1 oz	127	15	6
whole, salted; roasted	1 cup	285	34	12
whole; roasted	1 oz	127	15	6
whole; roasted	1 cup	285	34	12

PURSLANE

FRESH

FOOD	PORTION	CALORIES	CHO	FAT
cooked	1 cup	21	4	tr
raw	1 cup	7	1	tr

FOOD	PORTION	CALORIES	CHO	FAT
QUAIL				
breast w/o skin, raw	1 (2 oz)	69	0	2
w/ skin, raw	1 quail (3.8 oz)	210	0	13
w/o skin, raw	1 quail (3.2 oz)	123	0	4
QUICHE				
Lorraine (home recipe)	⅛ of 8″ pie	600	29	48
QUINCE				
fresh	1	53	14	tr
QUINOA				
quinoa	½ cup	318	59	5
RABBIT				
domestic, w/o bone, raw	1 oz	39	0	2
domestic, w/o bone; roasted	3 oz	131	0	5
wild, w/o bone, raw	1 oz	32	0	tr
wild, w/o bone; stewed	3 oz	147	0	3
RACCOON				
roasted	3 oz	217	0	12
RADISHES				
DRIED Chinese	½ cup	157	37	tr

FOOD	PORTION	CALORIES	CHO	FAT
daikon	½ cup	157	37	tr
white icicle, raw; sliced	1 (3½ oz)	14	3	tr
FRESH				
Chinese, raw	1 (12 oz)	62	14	tr
Chinese, raw; sliced	½ cup	8	2	tr
Chinese; sliced, cooked	½ cup	13	3	tr
daikon, raw	1 (12 oz)	62	14	tr
daikon, raw; sliced	½ cup	8	2	tr
daikon; sliced, cooked	½ cup	13	3	tr
red, raw	10	7	2	tr
red; sliced	½ cup	10	2	tr
white icicle, raw; sliced	½ cup	7	1	tr
SPROUTS				
raw	½ cup	8	1	tr

RAISINS

FOOD	PORTION	CALORIES	CHO	FAT
golden seedless	1 cup	437	115	1
seedless	1 cup	434	115	1
seedless	1 tbsp	27	7	tr

RASPBERRIES

FOOD	PORTION	CALORIES	CHO	FAT
CANNED				
*in heavy syrup	½ cup	117	30	tr
FRESH				
raspberries	1 cup	61	14	1
raspberries	1 pint	154	36	2

FOOD	PORTION	CALORIES	CHO	FAT
FROZEN				
*sweetened	1 cup	256	65	tr
*sweetened	1 pkg (10 oz)	291	74	tr
RELISH				
*cranberry orange	½ cup	246	64	tr
sweet	1 tbsp	20	5	tr
RHUBARB				
fresh	½ cup	13	3	tr
frzn	½ cup	60	3	tr
*frzn; as prep w/ sugar	½ cup	139	37	tr
RICE				
BROWN				
long-grain, raw	½ cup	340	71	3
long-grain; cooked	½ cup	109	23	tr
medium-grain, raw	½ cup	344	12	3
medium-grain; cooked	½ cup	109	23	tr
WHITE				
glutinous, raw	½ cup	341	75	tr
glutinous; cooked	½ cup	116	25	tr
long-grain, instant, dry	½ cup	182	40	tr
long-grain, instant; cooked	½ cup	80	17	tr
long-grain, parboiled, dry	½ cup	341	75	tr
long-grain, parboiled, cooked	½ cup	100	22	tr

FOOD	PORTION	CALORIES	CHO	FAT
long-grain, raw	½ cup	336	74	tr
long-grain; cooked	½ cup	131	28	tr
medium-grain, raw	½ cup	353	78	tr
medium-grain; cooked	½ cup	132	29	tr
short-grain, raw	½ cup	358	79	tr
short-grain; cooked	½ cup	133	29	tr
starch	3½ oz	343	85	0

ROCKFISH

FRESH
Pacific, raw	3 oz	80	0	1
Pacific; cooked	3 oz	103	0	2
Pacific; cooked	1 fillet (5.2 oz)	180	0	3

ROE

raw	1 oz	39	tr	2
raw	3 oz	119	1	5

ROLL

HOME RECIPE
dinner	1 (1.2 oz)	120	20	3

READY-TO-EAT
dinner	1 (1 oz)	85	14	2
frankfurter	1 (8/pkg)	115	20	2
hamburger	1 (8/pkg)	115	20	2
hard	1	155	30	2
submarine	1 (4.7 oz)	155	30	2

FOOD	PORTION	CALORIES	CHO	FAT
ROSE APPLE				
fresh	3½ oz	32	7	tr
ROSE HIP				
fresh	3½ oz	91	19	0
ROSELLE				
fresh	1 cup	28	6	tr
ROSEMARY				
dried	1 tsp	4	1	tr
ROUGHY				
FRESH				
orange, raw	3 oz	107	0	6
RUTABAGA				
cooked, mashed	½ cup	41	9	tr
raw; cubed	½ cup	25	6	tr
SABLEFISH				
raw	3 oz	166	0	13
SMOKED				
sablefish	1 oz	72	0	6
sablefish	3 oz	218	0	17
SAFFLOWER				
seeds, dried	1 oz	147	10	11

FOOD	PORTION	CALORIES	CHO	FAT

SAFFRON

saffron	1 tsp	2	tr	tr

SAGE

ground	1 tsp	2	tr	tr

SALAD

TAKE-OUT

tossed, w/o dressing	1½ cups	32	7	tr
tossed, w/o dressing	¾ cup	16	3	0
tossed, w/o dressing, w/ cheese & egg	1½ cups	102	5	6
tossed, w/o dressing, w/ chicken	1½ cups	105	4	2
tossed, w/o dressing, w/ pasta & seafood	1½ cups	380	32	21
tossed, w/o dressing, w/ shrimp	1½ cups	107	7	2

SALAD DRESSING

HOME RECIPE

French	1 tbsp	88	1	10
vinegar & oil	1 tbsp	72	tr	8

READY-TO-USE

blue cheese	1 tbsp	77	1	8
French	1 tbsp	67	3	6
Italian	1 tbsp	69	2	7
Russian	1 tbsp	76	2	8

FOOD	PORTION	CALORIES	CHO	FAT
sesame seed	1 tbsp	68	1	7
Thousand Island	1 tbsp	59	2	6
READY-TO-USE REDUCED CALORIE				
French	1 tbsp	22	4	1
Italian	1 tbsp	16	1	2
Russian	1 tbsp	23	5	1
Thousand Island	1 tbsp	24	3	2

SALMON

FOOD	PORTION	CALORIES	CHO	FAT
CANNED				
chum w/bone	3 oz	120	0	5
chum w/bone	1 can (13.9 oz)	521	0	20
pink w/bone	3 oz	118	0	5
pink w/bone	1 can (15.9 oz)	631	0	27
sockeye w/bone	3 oz	130	0	6
sockeye w/bone	1 can (12.9 oz)	566	0	27
FRESH				
Atlantic, raw	3 oz	121	0	5
Chinook, raw	3 oz	153	0	9
chum, raw	3 oz	102	0	3
coho, raw	3 oz	124	0	5
coho; cooked	3 oz	157	0	6
coho; cooked	½ fillet (5.4 oz)	286	0	12

FOOD	PORTION	CALORIES	CHO	FAT
pink, raw	3 oz	99	0	3
sockeye, raw	3 oz	143	0	7
sockeye; cooked	3 oz	183	0	9
sockeye; cooked	½ fillet (5.4 oz)	334	0	17
SMOKED				
Chinook	1 oz	33	0	1
Chinook	3 oz	99	0	4

SALSIFY

FRESH				
cooked, sliced	½ cup	46	10	tr
raw; sliced	½ cup	55	12	tr

SALT/SEASONED SALT

salt	1 tsp	0	0	0

SAPODILLA

fresh	1	140	34	2
fresh; cut up	1 cup	199	48	3

SAPOTES

fresh	1	301	76	1

SARDINES

CANNED				
Atlantic in oil w/ bone	1 can (3.2 oz)	192	0	11
Atlantic in oil w/ bone	2	50	0	3

FOOD	PORTION	CALORIES	CHO	FAT
Pacific in tomato sauce w/ bone	1 can (13 oz)	658	0	44
Pacific in tomato sauce w/ bone	1	68	0	5
FRESH				
raw	3½ oz	135	0	5

SAUCE

DRY				
bearnaise; as prep w/ milk & butter	1 cup	701	18	68
cheese; as prep w/ milk	1 cup	307	23	17
curry; as prep w/ milk	1 cup	270	26	15
mushroom; as prep w/ milk	1 cup	228	24	10
sour cream; as prep w/ milk	1 cup	509	45	30
stroganoff; as prep	1 cup	271	34	11
*sweet & sour; as prep	1 cup	294	73	tr
teriyaki; as prep	1 cup	131	28	1
white; as prep w/ milk	1 cup	241	21	13
JARRED				
barbecue	1 cup	188	32	5
teriyaki	1 tbsp	15	3	0
teriyaki	1 oz	30	6	0

SAUERKRAUT

CANNED				
sauerkraut	½ cup	22	5	tr

FOOD	PORTION	CALORIES	CHO	FAT
SAUSAGE				
blutwurst, uncooked	3½ oz	424	0	39
bockwurst, pork & veal, raw	1 link (2.3 oz)	200	tr	18
bockwurst, pork & veal, raw	1 oz	87	tr	8
bratwurst, pork; cooked	1 link (3 oz)	256	2	22
bratwurst, pork; cooked	1 oz	85	1	7
brotwurst, pork	1 oz	92	1	8
brotwurst, pork & beef	1 link (2.5 oz)	226	2	19
country-style pork; cooked	1 patty (1 oz)	100	tr	8
country-style pork; cooked	1 link (½ oz)	48	tr	4
gelbwurst, uncooked	3½ oz	363	0	33
Italian, pork, raw	1 (3 oz)	315	1	29
Italian, pork, raw	1 (4 oz)	391	1	35
Italian, pork; cooked	1 (2.4 oz)	216	1	17
Italian, pork; cooked	1 (3 oz)	268	1	21
kielbasa, pork	1 oz	88	1	8
knockwurst, pork & beef	1 (2.4 oz)	209	1	19
knockwurst, pork & beef	1 oz	87	1	8
mettwurst, uncooked	3½ oz	483	0	45
plockwurst, uncooked	3½ oz	312	0	45
Polish, pork	1 (8 oz)	739	4	65
Polish, pork	1 oz	92	tr	8
pork & beef; cooked	1 patty (1 oz)	107	1	10
pork & beef; cooked	1 link (½ oz)	52	tr	5
pork, raw	1 patty (2 oz)	238	1	23

FOOD	PORTION	CALORIES	CHO	FAT
pork, raw	1 link (1 oz)	118	tr	11
pork; cooked	1 patty (1 oz)	100	tr	8
pork; cooked	1 link (½ oz)	48	tr	4
Regensburger, uncooked	3½ oz	354	0	31
smoked, pork	1 link (2.4 oz)	256	1	22
smoked, pork	1 sm link (½ oz)	62	tr	5
smoked, pork & beef	1 link (2.4 oz)	229	1	21
smoked, pork & beef	1 sm link (½ oz)	54	tr	5
Vienna, canned	1 (½ oz)	45	tr	4
Vienna, canned	7 (4 oz)	315	2	28
weisswurst, uncooked	3½ oz	305	0	27
TAKE-OUT				
pork	1 patty (1 oz)	100	tr	8
pork	1 link (.5 oz)	48	tr	4

SAVORY

ground	1 tsp	4	1	tr

SCALLOP

FRESH				
raw	3 oz	75	2	1
HOME RECIPE				
breaded & fried	2 lg	67	3	3
TAKE-OUT				
breaded & fried	6 (5 oz)	386	38	19

FOOD	PORTION	CALORIES	CHO	FAT
SCUP				
FRESH				
raw	3 oz	89	0	2
SEAWEED				
DRIED				
agar	1 oz	87	23	tr
spirulina	1 oz	83	7	2
FRESH				
agar	1 oz	tr	2	tr
Irish moss	1 oz	14	4	tr
kelp	1 oz	12	3	tr
kombu	1 oz	12	3	tr
laver	1 oz	10	1	tr
nori	1 oz	10	1	tr
spirulina	1 oz	7	1	tr
tangle	1 oz	12	3	tr
wakame	1 oz	13	3	tr
SEMOLINA				
dry	½ cup	303	61	tr
SESAME				
seeds	1 tsp	16	tr	2
seeds, dried	1 tbsp	52	2	5
seeds, dried	1 cup	825	34	72
seeds, roasted & toasted	1 oz	161	7	14

FOOD	PORTION	CALORIES	CHO	FAT
sesame butter	1 tbsp	95	4	8
tahini from roasted & toasted kernels	1 tbsp	89	3	8
tahini from stone ground kernels	1 tbsp	86	4	7
tahini from unroasted kernels	1 tbsp	85	3	8

SESBANIA

flower	1	1	tr	0
flowers	1 cup	5	1	tr
flowers; cooked	1 cup	23	5	tr

SHAD

FRESH				
American, raw	3 oz	167	0	12

SHALLOTS

DRIED				
dried	1 tbsp	3	1	0
FRESH				
raw; chopped	1 tbsp	7	2	tr

SHARK

batter-dipped & fried	3 oz	194	5	12
raw	3 oz	111	0	4

FOOD	PORTION	CALORIES	CHO	FAT

SHEEPSHEAD FISH

FOOD	PORTION	CALORIES	CHO	FAT
cooked	1 fillet (6.5 oz)	234	0	3
cooked	3 oz	107	0	1
raw	3 oz	92	0	2

SHELLFISH SUBSTITUTES

FOOD	PORTION	CALORIES	CHO	FAT
crab, imitation	3 oz	87	1	1
scallop, imitation	3 oz	84	9	tr
shrimp, imitation	3 oz	86	8	1
surimi	1 oz	28	2	tr
surimi	3 oz	84	6	1

SHELLIE BEANS

FOOD	PORTION	CALORIES	CHO	FAT
CANNED				
shellie beans	½ cup	37	8	tr

SHRIMP

FOOD	PORTION	CALORIES	CHO	FAT
canned	1 cup	154	1	3
canned	3 oz	102	1	2
FRESH				
cooked	4 lg	22	0	tr
cooked	3 oz	84	0	1
raw	3 oz	90	1	1
raw	4 lg	30	tr	tr
HOME RECIPE				
breaded & fried	3 oz	206	10	10

FOOD	PORTION	CALORIES	CHO	FAT
breaded & fried	4 lg	73	3	4
TAKE-OUT				
breaded & fried	6 to 8 (6 oz)	454	40	25

SMELT

FRESH				
rainbow, raw	3 oz	83	0	2
rainbow; cooked	3 oz	106	0	3

SNAP BEANS

CANNED				
green	½ cup	13	3	tr
yellow	½ cup	13	3	tr
FRESH				
green, raw	½ cup	17	4	tr
green; cooked	½ cup	22	5	tr
yellow, raw	½ cup	17	4	tr
yellow; cooked	½ cup	22	5	tr
FROZEN				
cooked	½ cup	18	4	tr
yellow; cooked	½ cup	18	4	tr

SNAPPER

FRESH				
cooked	1 fillet (6 oz)	217	0	3
cooked	3 oz	109	0	1
raw	3 oz	85	0	1

FOOD	PORTION	CALORIES	CHO	FAT
SODA				
club	12 oz	0	0	0
*cola	12 oz	151	39	tr
*cream	12 oz	191	49	0
diet cola	12 oz	2	tr	0
diet cola w/ Nutrasweet	12 oz	2	tr	0
diet cola w/ saccharin	12 oz	2	tr	0
*ginger ale	12 oz	124	32	0
*grape	12 oz	161	42	0
*lemon lime	12 oz	149	38	0
*orange	12 oz	177	46	0
*pepper type	12 oz	151	38	tr
*quinine	12 oz	125	32	0
*root beer	12 oz	152	39	0
*tonic water	12 oz	125	32	0
SOLE				
FRESH				
lemon, raw	3½ oz	85	0	1
raw	3½ oz	90	0	1
SORGHUM				
sorghum	½ cup	325	72	3
SOUFFLÉ				
HOME RECIPE				
spinach soufflé	1 cup	218	3	18

FOOD	PORTION	CALORIES	CHO	FAT

SOUP

CANNED

FOOD	PORTION	CALORIES	CHO	FAT
asparagus, cream of; as prep w/ milk	1 cup	161	16	8
asparagus, cream of; as prep w/ water	1 cup	87	11	4
bean black; as prep w/ water	1 cup	116	20	2
beef broth, ready-to-serve	1 can (14 oz)	27	tr	1
beef broth, ready-to-serve	1 cup	16	tr	1
beef noodle; as prep w/ water	1 cup	84	9	3
celery, cream of; as prep w/ milk	1 cup	165	15	10
celery, cream of; as prep w/ water	1 cup	90	9	6
celery, cream of; not prep	1 can (10¾ oz)	219	21	14
cheese; as prep w/ milk	1 cup	230	16	15
cheese; as prep w/ water	1 cup	155	11	10
cheese; not prep	1 can (11 oz)	377	26	25
chicken vegetable; as prep w/water	1 cup	74	9	3
chicken broth; as prep w/ water	1 cup	39	1	1
chicken, cream of; as prep w/ milk	1 cup	191	15	11
chicken, cream of; as prep w/ water	1 cup	116	9	7

FOOD	PORTION	CALORIES	CHO	FAT
chicken gumbo; as prep w/ water	1 cup	56	8	1
chicken noodle; as prep w/ water	1 cup	75	9	2
chicken rice; as prep w/ water	1 cup	251	7	2
clam chowder, Manhattan; as prep w/ water	1 cup	78	12	2
clam chowder, New England; as prep w/ milk	1 cup	163	17	7
clam chowder, New England; as prep w/ water	1 cup	95	12	3
consommé w/ gelatin; as prep w/ water	1 cup	29	2	0
consommé w/ gelatin; not prep	1 can (10½ oz)	71	4	0
escarole, ready-to-serve	1 cup	27	2	2
French onion; as prep w/ water	1 cup	57	8	2
gazpacho, ready-to-serve	1 cup	57	1	2
minestrone; as prep w/ water	1 cup	83	11	3
mushroom, cream of; as prep w/ milk	1 cup	203	15	14
mushroom, cream of; as prep w/ water	1 cup	129	9	9
oyster stew; as prep w/ milk	1 cup	134	10	8
oyster stew; as prep w/ water	1 cup	59	4	4

FOOD	PORTION	CALORIES	CHO	FAT
pepperpot; as prep w/ water	1 cup	103	9	5
potato, cream of; as prep w/ milk	1 cup	148	17	6
potato, cream of; as prep w/ water	1 cup	73	11	2
Scotch broth; as prep w/ water	1 cup	80	9	3
split pea w/ ham; as prep w/ water	1 cup	189	28	4
tomato; as prep w/ milk	1 cup	160	22	6
tomato; as prep w/ water	1 cup	86	17	2
turtle bean	1 cup	218	40	1
vegetarian vegetable; as prep w/ water	1 cup	72	12	2
vichyssoise	1 cup	148	17	6
DRY				
asparagus, cream of; as prep w/ water	1 cup	59	9	2
beef broth; as prep w/ water	1 cup	19	2	1
beef broth; as prep w/water	1 cube + 1 cup water	8	1	tr
beef broth; not prep	1 pkg (.2 oz)	14	1	1
beef broth; not prep	1 cube (3.6 g)	6	1	tr
celery, cream of; as prep w/ water	1 cup	63	10	2
chicken broth cube; as prep w/ water	1 cup	13	2	tr

FOOD	PORTION	CALORIES	CHO	FAT
chicken broth; as prep w/ water	1 cup	21	1	1
chicken broth; not prep	1 pkg (.2 oz)	16	1	1
chicken broth; not prep	1 cube (4.8 g)	9	1	tr
chicken, cream of; as prep w/ water	1 cup	107	13	5
chicken noodle; as prep w/ water	1 cup	53	7	1
French onion; not prep	1 pkg (1.4 oz)	115	21	2
leek; as prep w/ water	1 cup	71	11	2
onion; as prep w/ water	1 cup	28	5	1
onion; not prep	1 pkg (1.4 oz)	115	21	2
tomato; as prep w/ water	1 cup	102	19	2
HOME RECIPE turtle bean soup	1 cup	241	45	1

SOUR CREAM

REGULAR

sour cream	1 tbsp	26	1	3
sour cream	1 cup	493	10	48

SOUR CREAM SUBSTITUTES

nondairy	1 oz	59	2	6
nondairy	1 cup	479	15	45

SOURSOP

fresh	1	416	105	2

FOOD	PORTION	CALORIES	CHO	FAT
fresh; cut up	1 cup	150	38	1

SOY

lecithin	1 tbsp	120	0	14
milk	1 cup	79	4	5
soy sauce	1 tbsp	7	1	tr
soy sauce, shoyu	1 tbsp	9	2	tr
soy sauce, tamari	1 tbsp	11	1	tr
soybean sprouts, raw	½ cup	45	4	2
soybean sprouts; cooked	½ cup	38	3	2
soybeans, dry roasted	½ cup	387	28	19
soybeans, roasted	½ cup	405	29	22
soybeans, roasted & toasted	1 oz	129	9	7
soybeans, roasted & toasted	1 cup	490	33	26
soybeans, salted, roasted & toasted	1 oz	129	9	7
soybeans, salted, roasted & toasted	1 cup	490	33	26
soybeans, dried	1 cup	774	56	37
soybeans; cooked	1 cup	298	17	15

SPAGHETTI SAUCE

JARRED
marinara sauce	1 cup	171	25	8
spaghetti sauce	1 cup	272	40	12

FOOD	PORTION	CALORIES	CHO	FAT

SPINACH

CANNED

| spinach | ½ cup | 25 | 4 | 1 |

FRESH

cooked	½ cup	21	3	tr
mustard, raw; chopped	½ cup	17	3	tr
mustard; chopped, cooked	½ cup	14	3	tr
New Zealand, raw	½ cup	4	1	tr
New Zealand; chopped, cooked	½ cup	11	2	tr
raw; chopped	½ cup	6	1	tr
raw; chopped	1 pkg (10 oz)	46	7	1

FROZEN

| cooked | ½ cup | 27 | 5 | tr |

JUICE

| spinach juice | 3½ oz | 7 | 1 | 0 |

SPOT

FRESH

| raw | 3 oz | 105 | 0 | 4 |

SQUAB

breast w/o skin, raw	1 (3.5 oz)	135	0	5
w/ skin, raw	1 squab (6.9 oz)	584	0	47
w/o skin, raw	1 squab (5.9 oz)	239	0	13

FOOD	PORTION	CALORIES	CHO	FAT
SQUASH				
CANNED				
crookneck; sliced	½ cup	14	3	tr
FRESH				
acorn; cooked, mashed	½ cup	41	11	tr
acorn; cubed, baked	½ cup	57	15	tr
butternut; baked	½ cup	41	11	tr
crookneck, raw; sliced	½ cup	12	3	tr
crookneck; sliced, cooked	½ cup	18	4	tr
hubbard; baked	½ cup	51	11	tr
hubbard; cooked, mashed	½ cup	35	8	tr
scallop, raw; sliced	½ cup	12	3	tr
scallop; sliced, cooked	½ cup	14	3	tr
spaghetti; cooked	½ cup	23	5	tr
FROZEN				
butternut; cooked, mashed	½ cup	47	12	tr
crookneck; sliced, cooked	½ cup	24	5	tr
SEEDS				
dried	1 oz	154	5	13
dried	1 cup	747	25	63
roasted	1 oz	148	4	12
roasted	1 cup	1184	31	96
salted & roasted	1 oz	148	4	12
salted & roasted	1 cup	1184	31	96
whole, salted; roasted	1 oz	127	15	6
whole, salted; roasted	1 cup	285	34	12

FOOD	PORTION	CALORIES	CHO	FAT
whole; roasted	1 oz	127	15	6
whole; roasted	1 cup	285	34	12

SQUID

FRESH

fried	3 oz	149	7	6
raw	3 oz	78	3	1

SQUIRREL

raw	1 oz	34	0	1
roasted	3 oz	116	0	3

STRAWBERRIES

CANNED

*in heavy syrup	½ cup	117	30	tr

FRESH

strawberries	1 cup	45	10	1
strawberries	1 pint	97	22	1

FROZEN

*sweetened sliced	1 cup	245	66	tr
*sweetened sliced	1 pkg (10 oz)	273	74	tr
unsweetened	1 cup	52	14	tr
*whole sweetened	1 cup	200	54	tr
*whole sweetened	1 pkg (10 oz)	223	60	tr

STUFFING/DRESSING

MIX

bread, dry	1 cup	500	50	31

FOOD	PORTION	CALORIES	CHO	FAT
STURGEON				
FRESH				
cooked	3 oz	115	0	4
raw	3 oz	90	0	3
SMOKED				
sturgeon	3 oz	147	0	4
sturgeon	1 oz	48	0	1
SUCKER				
FRESH				
white, raw	3 oz	79	0	2
SUGAR				
*brown	1 cup	820	212	0
*powdered; sifted	1 cup	385	100	0
*white	1 cup	770	199	0
*white	1 tbsp	45	12	0
*white	1 packet (6 g)	25	6	0
SUGAR APPLE				
fresh	1	146	37	tr
fresh; cut up	1 cup	236	59	1
SUNFISH				
FRESH				
pumpkinseed, raw	3 oz	76	0	1

FOOD	PORTION	CALORIES	CHO	FAT
SUNFLOWER SEEDS				
dried	1 oz	162	5	14
dried	1 cup	821	27	71
dry roasted	1 oz	165	7	14
dry roasted	1 cup	745	31	64
dry roasted, salted	1 oz	165	7	14
dry roasted, salted	1 cup	745	31	64
oil roasted	1 oz	175	4	16
oil roasted	1 cup	830	20	78
oil roasted, salted	1 cup	830	20	78
oil roasted, salted	1 oz	175	4	16
sunflower butter w/o salt	1 tbsp	93	4	8
toasted	1 oz	176	6	16
toasted	1 cup	826	28	76
toasted, salted	1 oz	176	6	16
toasted, salted	1 cup	826	28	76
SWAMP CABBAGE				
FRESH				
chopped, cooked	½ cup	10	2	tr
raw; chopped	1 cup	11	2	tr
SWEET POTATO				
CANNED				
*in syrup	½ cup	106	25	tr
pieces	1 cup	183	42	tr

FOOD	PORTION	CALORIES	CHO	FAT
FRESH				
baked w/ skin	1 (3½ oz)	118	28	tr
leaves; cooked	½ cup	11	2	tr
mashed	½ cup	172	40	tr
FROZEN				
cooked	½ cup	88	21	tr
HOME RECIPE				
*candied	3½ oz	144	29	3

SWEETBREADS

beef; braised	3 oz	230	0	15
lamb; braised	3 oz	199	0	13
veal; braised	3 oz	218	0	12

SWISS CHARD

FRESH				
cooked	½ cup	18	4	tr
raw; chopped	½ cup	3	1	tr

SWORDFISH

cooked	3 oz	132	0	4
raw	3 oz	103	0	3

SYRUP

*corn	2 tbsp	122	32	0
*raspberry	3½ oz	267	66	0

FOOD	PORTION	CALORIES	CHO	FAT
TAMARIND				
FRESH				
cut up	1 cup	287	75	1
tamarind	1	5	1	tr
TANGERINE				
CANNED				
*in light syrup	½ cup	76	20	tr
juice pack	½ cup	46	12	tr
FRESH				
sections	1 cup	86	22	tr
tangerine	1	37	9	tr
JUICE				
*canned sweetened	1 cup	125	30	1
fresh	1 cup	106	25	tr
*frzn sweetened, not prep	6 oz	344	83	1
*frzn sweetened; as prep	1 cup	110	27	tr
TAPIOCA				
pearl, dry	⅓ cup	174	45	0
starch	3½ oz	344	85	tr
TARO				
chips	10	110	15	6
chips	½ cup	57	8	3
leaves; cooked	½ cup	18	3	tr
raw; sliced	½ cup	56	14	tr

FOOD	PORTION	CALORIES	CHO	FAT
shoots; sliced, cooked	½ cup	10	2	tr
sliced, cooked	½ cup	94	23	tr
Tahitian; sliced, cooked	½ cup	30	5	tr

TARRAGON

ground	1 tsp	5	1	tr

TEA/HERBAL TEA

REGULAR

brewed tea	6 oz	2	tr	0
instant artificially sweetened, lemon flavored; as prep w/ water	8 oz	5	1	0
*instant sweetened, lemon flavor; as prep w/ water	9 oz	87	22	tr
instant unsweetened, lemon flavor; as prep w/ water	8 oz	4	0	0
instant unsweetened; as prep w/ water	8 oz	2	tr	0

TEMPEH

tempeh	½ cup	165	14	6

TEXTURED VEGETABLE PROTEIN

simulated meat product	1 oz	88	11	1

THYME

ground	1 tsp	4	1	tr

FOOD	PORTION	CALORIES	CHO	FAT
TILEFISH				
FRESH				
cooked	½ fillet (5.3 oz)	220	0	7
cooked	3 oz	125	0	4
raw	3 oz	81	0	2
TOFU				
firm	¼ block (3 oz)	118	3	7
fried	1 piece (½ oz)	35	1	3
fuyu, salted & fermented	1 block (⅓ oz)	13	1	1
koyadofu, dried, frozen	1 piece (½ oz)	82	2	5
okara	½ cup	47	8	1
regular	¼ block (4 oz)	88	2	6
TOMATO				
CANNED				
red, whole	½ cup	24	5	tr
stewed	½ cup	34	8	tr
tomato paste	½ cup	110	25	1
tomato paste w/o salt	½ cup	110	25	1
tomato puree	1 cup	102	25	tr
tomato puree w/o salt	1 cup	102	25	tr
tomato sauce	½ cup	37	9	tr
tomato sauce spanish style	½ cup	40	9	tr
tomato sauce w/ mushrooms	½ cup	42	10	tr

FOOD	PORTION	CALORIES	CHO	FAT
tomato sauce w/ onion	½ cup	52	12	tr
tomatoes w/ green chilies	½ cup	18	4	tr
wedges in tomato juice	½ cup	34	8	tr
FRESH				
cooked	½ cup	30	7	tr
green	1	30	6	tr
red	1	24	5	tr
red; chopped	1 cup	35	8	tr
HOME RECIPE				
stewed tomatoes	1 cup	59	10	2
JUICE				
beef broth & tomato	5½ oz	61	14	tr
clam & tomato	1 can (5½ oz)	77	18	tr
tomato juice	6 oz	32	8	tr
tomato juice	½ cup	21	5	tr

TONGUE

beef; simmered	3 oz	241	tr	18
lamb; braised	3 oz	234	0	17

TREE FERN

chopped, cooked	½ cup	28	8	tr

TRITICALE

dry	½ cup	323	69	2

FOOD	PORTION	CALORIES	CHO	FAT

TROUT

FRESH

FOOD	PORTION	CALORIES	CHO	FAT
rainbow, raw	3 oz	100	0	3
rainbow; cooked	3 oz	129	0	4
seatrout, raw	3 oz	88	0	3

TRUFFLES

FOOD	PORTION	CALORIES	CHO	FAT
fresh	3½ oz	25	17	1

TUNA

CANNED

FOOD	PORTION	CALORIES	CHO	FAT
light in oil	3 oz	169	0	7
light in oil	1 can (6 oz)	399	0	14
light in water	1 can (5.8 oz)	216	0	1
light in water	3 oz	111	0	tr
white in oil	3 oz	158	0	7
white in oil	1 can (6.2 oz)	331	0	14
white in water	1 can (6 oz)	234	0	4
white in water	3 oz	116	0	2

FRESH

FOOD	PORTION	CALORIES	CHO	FAT
bluefin, raw	3 oz	122	0	4
bluefin; cooked	3 oz	157	0	5
skipjack, raw	3 oz	88	0	1
yellowfin, raw	3 oz	92	0	1

FOOD	PORTION	CALORIES	CHO	FAT
TUNA DISHES				
TAKE-OUT				
tuna salad	3 oz	159	8	8
tuna salad	1 cup	383	19	19
tuna salad submarine sandwich w/ lettuce, oil	1	584	55	28
TURBOT				
FRESH				
European, raw	3 oz	81	0	3
TURKEY				
CANNED				
w/ broth	½ can (2.5 oz)	116	0	5
w/ broth	1 can (5 oz)	231	0	10
FRESH				
back w/ skin; roasted	½ back (9 oz)	637	0	38
breast w/ skin; roasted	4 oz	212	0	8
dark meat w/ skin; roasted	3.6 oz	230	0	12
dark meat w/o skin; roasted	3 oz	170	0	7
dark meat w/o skin; roasted	1 cup (5 oz)	262	0	10
leg w/ skin; roasted	2.5 oz	147	0	7
leg w/ skin; roasted	1 (1.2 lbs)	1133	0	54
light meat w/ skin; roasted	4.7 oz	268	0	11
light meat w/ skin; roasted	from ½ turkey (2.3 lbs)	2069	0	87

FOOD	PORTION	CALORIES	CHO	FAT
light meat w/o skin; roasted	4 oz	183	0	4
neck, raw	1 (6.3 oz)	243	0	10
neck; simmered	1 (5.3 oz)	274	0	11
skin; roasted	1 oz	141	0	13
skin; roasted	from ½ turkey (9 oz)	1096	0	98
w/ skin, neck & giblets, raw	½ turkey (6 lbs)	4369	2	216
w/ skin, neck & giblets, raw	9 oz	533	tr	25
w/ skin, neck & giblets; roasted	½ turkey (8.8 lbs)	4123	1	190
w/ skin; roasted	½ turkey (4 lbs)	3857	0	181
w/ skin; roasted	8.4 oz	498	0	23
w/o skin; roasted	7.3 oz	354	0	10
w/o skin; roasted	1 cup (5 oz)	238	0	7
wing w/ skin; roasted	1 (6.5 oz)	426	0	23
FROZEN roast, boneless, seasoned, light & dark meat, raw	1 pkg (2.5 lbs)	1358	73	25
roast, boneless, seasoned, light & dark meat; roasted	1 pkg (1.7 lbs)	1213	24	45
FROZEN PREPARED gravy & turkey	1 cup (8.4 oz)	160	11	6
gravy & turkey	1 pkg (5 oz)	95	7	4
READY-TO-USE bologna	1 oz	57	tr	4

FOOD	PORTION	CALORIES	CHO	FAT
breast	1 slice (¾ oz)	23	0	tr
diced, light & dark, seasoned	1 oz	39	tr	2
diced, light & dark, seasoned	½ lb	313	2	14
ham, thigh meat	2 oz	73	tr	3
ham, thigh meat	1 pkg (8 oz)	291	1	12
pastrami	2 oz	80	1	4
pastrami	1 pkg (8 oz)	320	4	14
patties; battered, fried	1 (3.3 oz)	266	15	17
patties; battered, fried	1 (2.3 oz)	181	10	12
patties; breaded, fried	1 (2.3 oz)	181	10	12
patties; breaded, fried	1 (3.3 oz)	266	15	17
poultry salad sandwich spread	1 tbsp	109	1	2
poultry salad sandwich spread	1 oz	238	2	4
prebasted breast w/ skin; roasted	1 breast (3.8 lbs)	2175	0	60
prebasted breast w/ skin; roasted	½ breast (1.9 lbs)	1087	0	30
prebasted thigh w/ skin; roasted	1 thigh (11 oz)	494	0	27
roll, light & dark meat	1 oz	42	1	2
roll, light meat	1 oz	42	2	2
salami, cooked	2 oz	111	tr	8
salami, cooked	1 pkg (8 oz)	446	1	31

FOOD	PORTION	CALORIES	CHO	FAT
turkey loaf, breast meat	2 slices (1.5 oz)	47	0	1
turkey loaf, breast meat	1 pkg (6 oz)	187	0	3
turkey sticks; battered, fried	1 stick (2.3 oz)	178	11	11
turkey sticks; breaded, fried	1 stick (2.3 oz)	178	11	11

TURMERIC

FOOD	PORTION	CALORIES	CHO	FAT
ground	1 tsp	8	1	tr

TURNIPS

CANNED

FOOD	PORTION	CALORIES	CHO	FAT
greens	½ cup	17	3	tr

FRESH

FOOD	PORTION	CALORIES	CHO	FAT
cooked, mashed	½ cup	21	6	tr
greens, raw; chopped	½ cup	7	2	tr
greens; chopped, cooked	½ cup	15	3	tr
raw; cubed	½ cup	18	4	tr

FROZEN

FOOD	PORTION	CALORIES	CHO	FAT
greens; cooked	½ cup	24	4	tr

TURTLE

FOOD	PORTION	CALORIES	CHO	FAT
raw	3½ oz	85	0	1

TUSK FISH

FOOD	PORTION	CALORIES	CHO	FAT
raw	3½ oz	79	0	tr

FOOD	PORTION	CALORIES	CHO	FAT

VEAL

FRESH

FOOD	PORTION	CALORIES	CHO	FAT
cubed, lean only, raw	1 oz	31	0	1
cutlet, lean only; braised	3 oz	172	0	4
cutlet, lean only; fried	3 oz	156	0	4
ground, raw	1 oz	41	0	2
ground; broiled	3 oz	146	0	6
loin chop w/ bone, lean & fat, raw	1 chop (4.4 oz)	204	0	11
loin chop w/ bone, lean & fat; braised	1 chop (2.8 oz)	227	0	14
loin chop w/ bone, lean only; braised	1 chop (2.4 oz)	155	0	6
shoulder w/ bone, lean only, braised	3 oz	169	0	5
sirloin w/ bone, lean & fat; roasted	3 oz	171	0	9
sirloin w/ bone, lean only; roasted	3 oz	143	0	5

VEGETABLES, MIXED

CANNED

FOOD	PORTION	CALORIES	CHO	FAT
mixed vegetables	½ cup	39	8	tr
peas & carrots	½ cup	48	11	tr
peas & onions	½ cup	30	5	tr
succotash	½ cup	102	23	1

FROZEN

FOOD	PORTION	CALORIES	CHO	FAT
mixed vegetables; cooked	½ cup	54	12	tr

FOOD	PORTION	CALORIES	CHO	FAT
peas & carrots; cooked	½ cup	38	8	tr
peas & onions; cooked	½ cup	40	8	tr
succotash; cooked	½ cup	79	17	1
HOME RECIPE				
succotash	½ cup	111	23	1
JUICE				
vegetable juice cocktail	6 oz	34	8	tr
vegetable juice cocktail	½ cup	22	6	tr

VENISON

raw	1 oz	34	0	1
roasted	3 oz	134	0	3

VINEGAR

cider	1 tbsp	tr	1	0

WAFFLES

HOME RECIPE				
waffle	7" diam	245	154	13
MIX				
as prep w/ egg & milk	1 waffle (2.6 oz)	205	27	8

WALNUTS

black, dried	1 oz	172	3	16
black, dried; chopped	1 cup	759	15	71
English, dried	1 oz	182	5	18
English, dried; chopped	1 cup	770	22	74

FOOD	PORTION	CALORIES	CHO	FAT

WATER CHESTNUTS

CANNED				
Chinese, sliced	½ cup	35	9	tr
FRESH				
sliced	½ cup	66	15	tr

WATERCRESS

| raw; chopped | ½ cup | 2 | tr | tr |

WATERMELON

cut up	1 cup	50	11	1
wedge	1/16	152	35	2
SEEDS				
dried	1 oz	158	4	13
dried	1 cup	602	17	51

WHALE

| raw | 3.5 oz | 134 | 0 | 3 |

WHEAT

| sprouted | 1/3 cup | 71 | 15 | tr |
| starch | 3½ oz | 348 | 86 | tr |

WHEAT GERM

| toasted | ¼ cup | 108 | 14 | 3 |
| untoasted | ¼ cup | 104 | 15 | 3 |

FOOD	PORTION	CALORIES	CHO	FAT
WHELK (SNAIL)				
FRESH				
cooked	3 oz	233	13	1
raw	3 oz	117	7	tr
WHIPPED TOPPINGS				
cream, pressurized	1 tbsp	8	tr	tr
cream, pressurized	1 cup	154	7	13
nondairy, powdered; as prep w/ whole milk	1 tbsp	8	1	tr
nondairy, powdered; as prep w/ whole milk	1 cup	151	13	10
nondairy, pressurized	1 tbsp	11	1	1
*nondairy, pressurized	1 cup	184	11	16
nondairy, frzn	1 tbsp	13	1	1
WHITE BEANS				
CANNED				
white beans	1 cup	306	58	1
DRIED				
regular, raw	1 cup	674	122	2
regular; cooked	1 cup	249	45	1
small, raw	1 cup	723	134	3
small; cooked	1 cup	253	46	1
WHITEFISH				
FRESH				
raw	3 oz	114	0	5

FOOD	PORTION	CALORIES	CHO	FAT
SMOKED				
whitefish	1 oz	39	0	tr
whitefish	3 oz	92	0	1

WHITING

FRESH				
cooked	3 oz	98	0	1
raw	3 oz	77	0	1

WILD RICE

cooked	½ cup	83	18	tr
raw	½ cup	286	60	tr

WINE

red	3½ oz	74	2	0
rose	3½ oz	73	2	0
*sweet dessert	2 oz	90	7	0
white	3½ oz	70	1	0

WINGED BEANS

DRIED				
cooked	1 cup	252	26	10
raw	1 cup	745	76	30

WOLFFISH

FRESH				
Atlantic, raw	3 oz	82	0	2

FOOD	PORTION	CALORIES	CHO	FAT

YAM

FOOD	PORTION	CALORIES	CHO	FAT
mountain yam, Hawaii; cooked	½ cup	59	14	tr
yam; cubed, cooked	½ cup	79	19	tr

YARDLONG BEANS

DRIED

FOOD	PORTION	CALORIES	CHO	FAT
cooked	1 cup	202	36	1
raw	1 cup	580	103	2

YEAST

FOOD	PORTION	CALORIES	CHO	FAT
baker's dry active	1 pkg (7 g)	20	3	tr
brewer's dry	1 tbsp	25	3	tr

YELLOW BEANS

DRIED

FOOD	PORTION	CALORIES	CHO	FAT
cooked	1 cup	254	45	2
raw	1 cup	676	119	5

YELLOWTAIL

FRESH

FOOD	PORTION	CALORIES	CHO	FAT
raw	3 oz	124	0	4

YOGURT

FOOD	PORTION	CALORIES	CHO	FAT
*coffee, lowfat	8 oz	194	31	3
*fruit, lowfat	4 oz	113	21	1
*fruit, lowfat	8 oz	225	42	3
plain	8 oz	139	11	7

FOOD	PORTION	CALORIES	CHO	FAT
plain, lowfat	8 oz	144	16	4
plain, no fat	8 oz	127	17.	tr
*vanilla, lowfat	8 oz	194	31	3

ZUCCHINI

CANNED
| Italian style | ½ cup | 33 | 8 | tr |

FRESH
| raw; sliced | ½ cup | 9 | 2 | tr |
| sliced, cooked | ½ cup | 14 | 4 | tr |

FROZEN
| cooked | ½ cup | 19 | 4 | tr |

INDEX

(HB) = Highlight Box

THE
SUPERMARKET
NUTRITION
COUNTER

BE A SAVVY SHOPPER WITH
MONEY-SAVING, HEALTH-CONSCIOUS
TIPS FROM TWO NATIONALLY
RECOGNIZED NUTRITION EXPERTS

OVER 16,000 ITEMS

Annette Natow, Ph.D.,R.D., and Jo-Ann Heslin, M.A.,R.D.

Bestselling Authors of
The Fat Counter* and *The Cholesterol Counter

POCKET
BOOKS

Available from Pocket Books

1076

THE
IRON COUNTER

**MONITOR YOUR IRON INTAKE
AND REDUCE YOUR RISK OF
HEART DISEASE**

**OVER 8,000 ENTRIES IDENTIFYING
KEY SOURCES OF IRON IN BRAND
NAME, GENERIC, AND FAST FOODS**

Annette Natow, Ph.D.,R.D.,
and Jo-Ann Heslin, M.A.,R.D.

**Bestselling Authors of
The Fat Counter and *The Cholesterol Counter***

POCKET
BOOKS

Available from Pocket Books

647-01